VOICE
LESSONS

Praise for *Voice Lessons*

"As one of the most gifted, prolific, and beloved actors in animation, it's no surprise that Rob Paulsen's book is fascinating, hugely entertaining, and laugh-out-loud funny. What I wasn't expecting was his candid, inspirational, and ultimately life-affirming account of facing devastating medical issues with such optimism, courage, and determination. I only regret I'm too old to play him in the inevitable movie version."

— Mark Hamill

"Rob is more than relentlessly optimistic, he is a disciplined professional, skilled in the art of positivity. Every session with Rob is a master class in technique and collegiality. It is a privilege to work with him. It is an honor to know him. If I could design a humanitarian award in the world of voice acting, I'd call it the Rob and make it a statue of him with a mic sticking out of his head. And the first Rob goes to...Rob."

— Sean Astin

"Having worked with Rob I knew of the deep well of talent he could draw upon to create the extraordinary range of characters from *Animainiacs*, to Pinky, to a couple of Ninja Turtles. But it isn't until someone is forced to confront their own mortality that you truly see their mettle. In watching Rob fight his way back to life, I discovered he is a treasure."

— Kevin Conroy

"Want to know about the world of voiceover from a professional? One who has acted in some of the best-known cartoons ever made? An actor who has been in demand for decades and has the respect of his peers? How about learning by example to face adversity and yet be triumphant? Then this is the book for you."
— Andrea Romano, Emmy award-winning casting and voice director

"One of the most accomplished and beloved performers in animation, Rob doesn't shy from shameless expression. In this memoir he goes even deeper, sharing his most personal struggles and discoveries along the way. It's a celebration of entertainment and the way it connects us all. It's an inspiring peek behind the magic, exposing the rawness of a performer's needs, the fears and insecurity we all share. He shines so brightly, it's like a lighthouse guiding your way on a journey you'll be glad you took."
— Seth Green

"I was stunned when I found out Rob had throat cancer. But true to form, he has NEVER been a victim. This page-turner will captivate and amaze you about the human spirit. Rob kills it, like his thousands of characters."

— Nancy Cartwright

"Rob Paulsen is inspirational to me not only for his legendary characters and ginormous heart, but now also for his incredible tale of strength and survival. I love this man!!! Cancer can go narf itself."

— Chris Hardwick

"Man, does Rob have skills! I was filled with joy the first time I ever worked with the guy. His story is also one of bravest I've ever known, because he battled back so valiantly from cancer."

— Billy West

"One of the most iconic, versatile, recognizable and hard-working voices in this industry, Rob has undoubtedly brought his magic through the world of animation, to the world of real life. He is truly one of the kindest, most inspiring and deeply connected individuals you will ever meet. I get the honor of working with him consistently, and he has without a doubt changed my performances as a voice actress forever. Out of all the many voices that he has portrayed, it is his own that has been the greatest gift to this world."

— Kat Graham

"*Pinky and The Brain* fans love to debate about which one is the genius and which one's insane. But as the guy who has shared a microphone with him for many years, I can tell you that in real life, Rob Paulsen is the genius, not only by virtue of his quick, facile mind and legendary skills behind the mic, but of his huge and open heart. As for this book, you'll find that, while you're enjoying what starts out as a fun and informative peek behind the curtain into our world, an honest tale of real courage, inner strength, and the redemptive power of human connection sneaks up on you, moves you to your core, and has you hooked to the very last page. While Brain may never admit to loving Pinky, I'm totally unashamed to proclaim, I LOVE ROB PAULSEN. You will, too."

— Maurice LaMarche a.k.a. The Brain

"Since I was a kid, I've had the pleasure of working with Rob on various animated projects, and I have always learned from watching him work. Now in this latest work, *Voice Lessons*, I have learned about living optimism. After decades of being entertained by the voices of his beloved characters, it's a privilege to experience this candid story told in his own authentic and hilarious voice. As well as being a top-notch entertainer, Rob is a lover of life and a champion of living at your best. Typical of anything that Rob creates, his positivity soars beyond the expected and into a do or die optimism that inspires, uplifts, and dares us all to be better."

— Scott Menville, *Teen Titans, Teen Titans Go!*

VOICE LESSONS

How a Couple of Ninja Turtles, Pinky, and an Animaniac Saved My Life

ROB PAULSEN

with *Michael Fleeman*

VIVA
EDITIONS

Published in the United States by Viva Editions, an imprint of Start Midnight, LLC, 101 Hudson Street, Thirty-Seventh Floor, Suite 3705, Jersey City, NJ 07302.

Printed in the United States.
Cover design: Allyson Fields
Cover image: Lesley Bohm
Text design: Frank Wiedemann

First Edition.
10 9 8 7 6 5 4 3 2 1

Trade paper ISBN: 978-1-63228-066-4
E-book ISBN: 978-1-63228-122-7

TABLE OF CONTENTS

This book is dedicated to the human spirit. It sounds a bit pretentious for a cartoon voice guy's story but the examples of utter courage in the everyday heroes cited herein have been and continue to be a source of inspiration, kindness, hope and faith for me. Family, friends and fans: We all fit those categories and we truly are all in this together, kids. So if my story inspires positive action, elicits joy, gives the reader strength . . . well, that, I believe, is what we're all here to do for each other. Narf.

Thank you, Parri, Ash, Pooshie, and Tala.
For making me a lottery winner. ♥

"Laughter's the best medicine:
the cool thing is, you can't OD and the refills are free."

FOREWORD

If a couple of Ninja Turtles, Pinky, and an Animaniac saved my dad's life, then it's fair to say mine has been heavily informed by the experience of growing up amid these and other colorful, unique characters.

I was surprised and a little confused at first when my dad asked me to write the foreword for this book. "Why not any number of the other world-class voice actors who were at once mutually talented colleagues and lifelong friends?" I wondered. I've been around for most of his voice acting career, of course, but other than a really exciting video game role he landed in the early aughts—whereas my dad has made his home and livelihood in the animation world, mine is firmly entrenched in the console gaming space—I've rarely found myself in the position of informing it. (That role was Gray Fox in *Metal Gear Solid: The Twin Snakes*, if you're wondering.)

But I soon realized that was exactly why: none of his colleagues have the unique perspective, at least as far as I'm aware, of knowing what it's like to grow up as the son of a world-class voice actor who has brought to aural life some of the most beloved, celebrated cartoon characters of all time. As you might imagine, that kind of career success, life fulfillment, and general notoriety can cast a large, looming shadow for a kid and, later, teenager and young adult trying to find their own place in the world.

But I would later realize, from a more adult perspective, that the whole gamut of experiences I had growing up amid my dad's work—especially the many positively great ones, like the nationwide trips for Warner Bros. Studio Store appearances I accompanied him for, or counting legends like Mark Hamill among the invitees to one of my birthday parties—were all fully contextualized by my dad's successes, not his failures. Much like how people today filter their lives on social media, I only ever saw the good aspects of his career; never the bad.

It wasn't until later on, as an adult having adult conversations with my dad, that I would be exposed to the other side of any successful career: his struggles, his disappointments, his failures. As Thanos said: "Perfectly balanced, as all things should be."

Fortunately, dear Rob Paulsen fan—which I imagine you must be if you're holding this book in your hands—you don't have to wait that long to learn about the full spectrum of my dad's career, and you don't even have to be related to him. The good and the bad, the moments on top of the world and at rock bottom; it's all here, set against the backdrop of the many and wide-ranging "voice lessons" he has learned throughout his career, many—if not most—tough and not so fun to learn.

But more importantly than a blow-by-blow account of my dad's life and career—and I do mean *blow-by-blow*, like this thing is astonishingly detailed—you'll learn what it means to leverage your own voice lessons in service of the voiceless, those whose lives have been beset by tragedy many of us can't even fathom, and those for whom meeting the voice behind a couple of Ninja Turtles, Pinky, and an Animaniac may well be one of the most important, exciting moments of their lives.

That's the one thing I hope you take away from this book, other than the kind of granular knowledge about my dad that would be right at home on a Trivial Pursuit card. Inspired by the utmost respect and humility with which my dad has always approached and treated his fans, I in turn have been fortunate enough in my adult life to have had the opportunity to carve out my own relatively public platform, which I have been able to use in service of bringing that same kind of goodness and humility to the fans I am fortunate enough to have in the gaming space.

Not everyone is lucky or privileged enough to have the chance to genuinely affect others' lives for the better, and too many of us who are simply don't, choosing instead to focus on the power and leverage their fame affords them over others. Over the course of reading *Voice Lessons*, I learned a lot of stuff about my dad's life and career that I never knew, and rest assured you will learn even more. And you, as a Rob Paulsen fan, will undoubtedly soak up every word of that stuff. But that's not what this book is really about. The real story, the real take-aways, are between the front-facing factoids about my dad's time on this planet—they are, in fact, found within the voice lessons we can all apply in our own lives to make the world a little better than it is today.

—Ash Paulsen

INTRODUCTION

Pinky Gets Bad News

"Pinky, I gotta tell you, dude. I got some bad news."

"Is it really bad, Rob?"

"Yeah, it's pretty bad. Maybe you can guess what it is?"

"Oh no. Wait a minute. Rosie O'Donnell is back on network TV?"

"No."

"I'm soaking in it?"

"No."

"Oh, you got me all freaked out, Rob. You've got me all . . ."

"Take a breath."

"Okay."

"Let's put it this way. I'm a Pisces, not a Cancer, although it seems I have it."

"You what? You have cancer? Are you going to die?"

"Well, I suppose I could. I don't really know yet."

"Well, who's gonna pay for this car?"

"You don't drive."

"Yeah, but you do, you idiot—and they call me the dumb one! Don't you die on me, I need food pellets—and maybe even a reboot someday."

I can talk to Pinky all day. I have a comfortable enough knowledge of the way he pronounces words, the phrases he would use, the ways he interacts with other characters—and human beings—that my brain shuts down and Pinky takes over. Rob checks out, and Pinky checks in.

I was lucky enough to "help create" him. I made a choice to have him struggle pronouncing Rs because of his buckteeth. I threw in a goofy kind of Cockney thing because Peter Sellers and *Monty Python's Flying Circus* were huge inspirations to me as a kid.

I say help create because there's so much more to Pinky. I often tell people: I don't draw 'em, I don't write 'em, I don't animate 'em.

I'm just the actor. I'm only as good as the concept and the writing and the direction, among many other factors. It takes an army of talented people and a series of happy (and sometimes painful) accidents to bring a character to life.

If you're really lucky, and lightning strikes, you end up with a character who doesn't just live but who becomes iconic.

In my case, I've been very lucky. Of the thousand or so characters I've voiced in more than thirty years of animation, I've been fortunate to boast of at least five that have occupied prominent places in pop culture: Pinky and Yakko from *Animaniacs*, Carl Wheezer from *Jimmy Neutron: Boy Genius*, and two Teenage Mutant Ninja Turtles, Raphael from the original show, and Donatello from a later version.

These characters have given me endless joy. I don't just voice them for money. No matter where I am—the store, the airport, even the cancer ward—it takes little prompting for me to whip them out. Then I watch as the joy I feel spreads. Children and adults, cops and nurses and soldiers and salespeople and lawyers, they can't help but smile and laugh.

Cartoon characters bring them back to a place of innocence and pure, unadulterated happiness. They're back in their living rooms, home from school, homework stuffed in their backpacks, maybe something cooking in the kitchen, and the TV tuned to their favorite shows.

And maybe now they have kids of their own, sharing a few minutes in front of the television, or more likely the computer or iPad, revisiting those wonderful cartoons, returning to a place so gentle and sweet, now laughing at the subversive jokes and sight gags they didn't get when they were kids.

There are a lot of reasons I wanted to write this book. One is I hoped that people would learn a little more about the actors behind those voices. For generations they brought nothing but happiness to the world, yet they worked in relative obscurity, performing their magic anonymously behind the microphone in recording studios in nondescript buildings in Burbank and Studio City.

The people who primarily work with their voices are among the most gifted, unpretentious, fearless actors I've known. Thanks to social media and the popularity of conventions like Comic-Con, we are finally more recognizable than we used to be. I would love for this book to shine an even brighter light on them.

I also want to show, in my little way, the hidden power of these cartoon characters. They make us giggle, of course, but it goes deeper. I've been fortunate enough to get to know countless children with serious health problems, many of them life-threatening. Brave kids like my buddy Chad, whom you'll meet later in this book. I talk to them in cartoon voices, sign posters, share a laugh and a hug and, often with their parents, tears. I always marvel at how much a few words from a Turtle can mean to a kid enduring circumstances none of us can imagine.

These moments so inspired me that I had considered writing this book years ago. Then one day, a little lump on my neck appeared. Without a brutal assault of radiation and chemicals, that lump would kill me, the doctors said. I was fortunate enough to live in an era in which modern science could cure me. By cure, I mean get rid of the lump. But would I be the same again? The doctors minced no words. They could cure me, but they couldn't guarantee that my voice would survive. I'd be able to speak, they said. But make a living as a voice actor? Their job, they said, was to save me, not my career.

And so I found myself at home one day lying in front of the TV, watching something on DVD, zonked on Vicodin or medicinal marijuana, my throat on fire, my stomach resistant to food and even water, dry heaving, manically hiccuping, wasting away. I looked in the mirror. A skeleton looked back with glassy eyes.

I'd become one of those sick kids I used to visit. I didn't feel sorry for myself. I didn't feel betrayed by my body. I didn't say, "Why me?" In fact, I usually said, "Why not me?" I'd had a marvelous life, lived every dream I had as a kid in Grand Blanc, Michigan. I was sixty years old. If I never worked another day in Hollywood again, well, so be it. If I were in corporate America, I might have been downsized by now anyway.

My story, I believe, is pretty small potatoes in terms of an actual physical struggle. But I learned a few lessons along the way that I hope will help others, lessons about faith and love and empathy, about growing older in an industry that craves youth, about what it means to almost lose everything you hold dear, only to discover those things that are the most important.

It's a story about how silence helped me speak louder than ever.

And it's about Pinky and Yakko and Carl and Raphael and Donatello and all those little critters banging around inside my head. It's about unleashing the power of humor and cartoons.

It's about Turtle Power, which, I'm proud to say, is very real.

CHAPTER ONE

A Kick in the Reboot

So three cartoon characters and a musician walk into a restaurant.

Morton's The Steakhouse, in Burbank, is down the street from the Warner Bros. lot, where Yakko, Wakko, and Dot Warner made their home in the water tower. A big dinner was set for this night, an honest-to-goodness Hollywood power meal, hosted by the big cheese at Warner Bros. for the benefit of three cartoon characters and a musician: myself, Jess Harnell, Tress MacNeille, and Randy Rogel—respectively Yakko, Wakko, Dot, and the primary songwriter from *Animaniacs*.

It was March of 2016, and naturally we were the noisiest table in the joint, a gaggle of artists with stunted emotional growth and little impulse control who make their living amusing your children when you're not looking, and sometimes when you are.

Morton's is one of those restaurants that has movie star pictures all over the walls. Bob Hope watched over us as we waited for Sam Register, the head of animation. We were chittering and chattering and making silly sounds. We gossiped and talked shop and caught up with each other. We've known each other for years, and we somehow all managed to keep working and, more importantly, remain the biggest friends in this crazy competitive business.

I put "actor" on my tax form. I don't necessarily delineate "voice actor" unless somebody says, "Have you ever done any real acting?"

Well . . . I guest starred as a junior G-man on *MacGyver,* played a husband on *New Love, American Style,* brought a friend into *St. Elsewhere,* and traveled through time in *Amazing Stories.* In the movies I played a porno film director and a gay flight attendant. In commercials I sold soft drinks, blue jeans, fried chicken, milk, and Hondas.

And if I still get a blank and disappointed look, I give 'em a little Pinky or Yakko or Carl or a Turtle. Then they know who I am.

This night, I had been a cartoon voice actor since the mid-1980s, when I baked up a Boston accent for a redheaded soldier named Snow Job for the first cartoon of *G.I. Joe.* That was back when Marvel was just making comic books and cartoons and not blockbusters starring Robert Downey Jr. in flying suits.

I've done over two thousand half hours of animation, and probably eleven hundred commercials. My IMDb page stretches from here to Mars with cartoon credits, volume always being the key to my career success. This is just voice work, specifically. I don't know how many video games, features, or direct-to-video things I've done.

Animaniacs is the big one. It changed my life. It still changes my life, the most precious professional gift I've ever received.

Now there were rumblings it was coming back.

Created by Tom Ruegger and executive produced by Steven Spielberg, the show ran for six seasons from 1993 to 1998, a delightful romp about three cartoon characters drawn originally back in the 1930s by the same folks at Warner Bros. Animation who came up with *Looney Tunes.* Wakko, Yakko, and Dot were deemed too irreverent, too difficult to handle, and thus got stashed in the water tower to keep them from getting into mischief. They were forgotten for decades until they ultimately escaped. Hilarity ensued.

The show took the form of a variety program, a sort of animated *Carol Burnett Show.* Yakko, Wakko, and Dot would sing and dance and star in comedy bits. They also introduced other segments, including some featuring another voice I do, a lab mouse named Pinky, who teamed with fellow mouse The Brain in his schemes for world domination, which inevitably fell flat. Their sequences became so popular they got their own show, *Pinky and the Brain.*

For two decades, fans had been asking if *Animaniacs* could ever come back on the air. It's one of the most common questions I get on

Twitter or at conventions. As *Animaniacs* survived and thrived in syndication and then on Netflix, the kids who watched it in the '90s started having their own kids.

Which we all figured explained this night's dinner. Reboot fever had been sweeping Hollywood and had spilled into animation. The reality was that none of us from the show had any better idea if the show was coming back than the average fan. We left *Animaniacs* with fond memories and fatter bank accounts and moved on to new voices.

But there were clues. A little more than two years before the Morton's dinner, Randy and I had approached Warner Bros. about securing the music license for a live stage show featuring *Animaniacs* songs. One of the singular joys of *Animaniacs* was that it allowed me to not only talk in character, but to sing.

The very first tune Randy Rogel wrote for the show was for my character: "Yakko's World," a rat-a-tat recitation of country names to the tune of the "Mexican Hat Dance." It immediately became an audience favorite and has been one of the reasons people still come to see me at comic conventions and live shows all these years later. It's my "My Way."

We were working up a show with Randy at the piano and me at the microphone, both of us singing his amazingly clever and catchy songs, sometimes synching the words to cartoon clips. We had a handshake deal on the rights. We wanted to make it all legal. For that we needed permission from Warner Bros. and Mr. Spielberg.

That's how, fifteen years after the show went off the air, Randy and I found ourselves in an office on the studio lot one day, schmoozing with the suits.

We were in one gentleman's office and had another muckety-muck on the line in New York. I was making the pitch, and things didn't seem to be going well. The guy in New York didn't seem to understand why I wanted to do this show with Randy.

About fifteen minutes into the conversation, the New York guy stopped in the middle of the meeting and said, "Wait a minute, Rob. Are you the guy who did the voices?"

"Yeah," I said.

"Oh my god. Now it makes sense."

With all the usual studio turnover, nobody knew who the hell we were. I looked at Randy and we could read each other's thoughts: *We're screwed.*

Warner Bros. kicked the idea around and so, I'm presuming, did Mr. Spielberg and his people, and in the end we got a great licensing deal. That allowed us to take the show all over the country, sometimes Randy on the piano and me singing, sometimes accompanied by full symphony orchestras. Audiences love it, and we have the best time doing it.

I began to suspect that one of the reasons Randy and I got the rights was because Warner Bros. and Spielberg were thinking of using our little performances as trial balloons to see if there was still a fan base for *Animaniacs.* It didn't escape our notice that at one of our bigger shows the audience was sprinkled with Warner Bros. brass.

And now here we were at Morton's, and Sam Register was taking his seat. After exchanging hellos, Sam got down to it: "Steven has been kicking around the idea of doing *Animaniacs* again."

Sam spoke of his respect for us and respect for the fan base and how they didn't want to make any mistakes. He very politely noted that we were getting a bit older and might be planning on retiring. He said that Steven—he calls him Steven; I'm still more comfortable with Mr. Spielberg—had made it clear that it was going to be with us four or he wouldn't do it at all.

"The bottom line is," Sam concluded, "would you guys be interested?"

He barely got this out of his mouth when we all lost our respective shit. Metaphorically, of course. This was a high-class restaurant.

That got a smile from Sam. "I kind of figured you'd say that," he said. "Trust me, the thought is very appealing to a lot of us."

We were all, of course, completely flattered and thrilled at being buttered up and told how important the voice actors are to the studio and to the fans. You have to understand, voice actors don't usually get the star treatment. We're paid well, treated professionally, and to a person we love our jobs with all our hearts, but let's face it, we're no Brad Pitts. No paparazzi wait outside Spago to get a shot of the guy who's a singing bacon strip on *VeggieTales.*

This potential reboot was a Big Deal involving Big Bucks. We're not talking about some goofy little show or a weird video game and somebody with a bunch of money thinking, "Hey, let's try to make this into a cartoon and find that old guy who did Pinky. Oh, it's Ron Pullman, or Rod . . . whoever he is."

We're talking about *Animaniacs* and Steven Spielberg, Warner Bros.—all of that.

We asked Sam how soon this would happen.

"We're not sure," Sam said. "We're on Steven time."

He chuckled, and we knew what he meant. Steven Spielberg is the king of Hollywood. He'll do it when he does it.

So we left the dinner very excited. In the parking lot, the four of us were glowing from flattery.

Then my stomach sank. Could it be true? Could they really be getting the old gang back together? None of us was getting younger. What a way to cap off a career. But it brought up conflicted emotions.

The good news was the studio wanted to do this.

The bad news was they wanted to do this.

It was all for one and one for all, and I didn't know if I was going to be one of those ones. I didn't know if I'd have any voice left when they got around to making the show. Hell, I didn't know if I'd have any me left.

"Guys," I said to my friends. "I haven't told Sam."

I was shaving one day in early 2015 when I found the lump on the left side of my neck. It was about a half an inch long, under my skin, very hard to the touch. I knew enough about basic anatomy to guess this was in the area of the lymph node. I figured it was swollen because of a bacterial infection. It would go away.

I didn't go to the doctor. For a fifty-nine-year-old, I felt like my health was great. I didn't smoke. I drank maybe twice a week, and then only a glass. I wasn't losing weight. I was playing golf two or three days a week. My prostate received regular visits by the doctor and cheerily responded with great PSA tests. I was working like crazy.

But I was just concerned enough to do some home research. Into Google I entered "swollen glands" and "swollen bump on neck." Back came everything from low-grade infection to impending slow and painful death. The testimonials on the cancer message boards offered massive doses of TMI, but also enough case studies that I could pick and choose so that I could focus on the good stuff and ignore the bad.

I could barely see the lump. I didn't tell any of my friends or work colleagues. I didn't tell my wife. One reason was I didn't want to worry her. The other reason was I didn't want her to say, "Honey, go get it looked at right now."

I am, for better or worse, a hopeless optimist, a glass-half-full kind of guy. In this case it was a little bit for worse. I ignored the lump.

My first voice lesson: my wife was right. I was an idiot.

In February 2016 I had an appointment at my internist's office to get a blood test in preparation for my annual physical. I felt great. I bounded into his offices in the Century City Medical Towers.

In the previous few years, I'd bounced back from the worst crisis of my professional life, one that had left me unemployed and put my marriage and sanity on the brink (we'll get to this later), and I was now busier than ever with both cartoon projects and my own endeavors.

I was working on the fifth season of *Teenage Mutant Ninja Turtles* as well as *The Fairly OddParents* for Nickelodeon. I was working on a show called *Doc McStuffins* for Disney TV, which would win another Peabody Award. I was doing live appearances. I had conventions booked throughout the year. My *Talkin' Toons* podcast was building an audience.

Life was good, and I like good. I come from cartoons, remember, where there's nothing that can't be solved with a big wooden mallet and a crate of Acme dynamite. It's not that I'm irresponsible, per se. Had one of my sports cars made a weird noise, I would have taken that bad boy to the dealership immediately and hooked it up to every scope in the garage. Had it been my wife or my son or my best friend, I would have dropped everything and done anything to help. It's only when trouble looms for me, personally, that I tend to catch the first boat to denial isle and find that sunny spot until the clouds pass.

So I wasn't particularly concerned that day when I took a seat in the waiting room. A couple minutes later, my internist happened to walk by. I wasn't supposed to see him for another few days for the physical. I don't know what prompted me, but I blurted out, "Hey, Doc, hang on a second. Would you do me a favor and just put your hands on this?"

I pointed to the lump.

He said, "Come on in the office."

Five seconds was all it took—five seconds for him to feel my neck and say, "Not good, Rob."

"Yeah, yeah, yeah," I said. Doc Paulsen, Google MD.

"No, seriously. This is not good. If it were an infection, it would be soft and pliable like it was filled with fluid," he said. "This is a knot. And it is a lymph node, not a gland. You need to see an ear, nose, and throat guy like yesterday."

I asked him what it could be.

"I'm not going to tell you too much, because you need to see an ENT and you've got to get a biopsy," he said. "If it's bad news, it'll probably be quite treatable, but you need to get right on this."

He arranged for an appointment with a specialist at Cedars-Sinai Medical Center in Beverly Hills—the hospital to the stars, and me. I maintained my usual positive Toontown attitude, happy as one of my cartoon alter egos.

I called my wife, Parrish, from the car and said there was something I needed to talk about.

"What?" she said, concerned. "Is it bad?"

"Well, maybe," I said.

"Is it Ashton?" she asked. Ash is our son.

"I have this lump," I said. "I didn't want to tell you anything until I knew more because it may be nothing, but I'm going to see a specialist in a couple days and I may be wearing a Band-Aid on my neck afterward, so you're going to say, 'What the hell happened?'"

She was not happy. Not for the first time, she reminded me I was an idiot. She usually says it with a big smile: "He's an idiot, but he's my idiot." My wife has to be understanding to be able to live with someone who does what I do for a living. Sometimes it has its advantages. She's from North Carolina, and one time when she went home to visit relatives—this was right around the time *Ninja Turtles* took off in the early '90s—she went to a drugstore in Shelby, North Carolina, to cash a check. But she forgot her ID, and the cashier wouldn't do it. The manager came out and recognized my name on the check.

"Go ahead," he said. "Her husband's Raphael. Turtles are good for the money."

On the other hand, I can't count how many times she's rolled her eyes at me. Typically this happens when we're in public and I find myself falling into character, often loudly, often surrounded by people, usually at inappropriate times. As you'll see, it doesn't take much for me to launch into a character. An appreciative fan. Sunlight. I'm a performer, I can't help it. Put the default setting on happy.

It took me a few days to get in to see the ear, nose, and throat doctor, more because of my schedule than his. I had a couple of cartoon gigs and I didn't want to turn down any work. The last thing I wanted to do was announce to Hollywood, "Hire me. But first I've got to see a guy about something growing on my neck."

It's no news flash that it's tough to grow old gracefully in Hollywood. Even in voice acting, in which nobody knows what you look like, ageism poses a real threat. I could see my career slipping back to the lonely, awful place I had just emerged from.

Luckily, one of the first lessons you learn in the talking business is knowing when to shut up.

In a week I saw the Cedars doctor. His walls were covered in plaques and diplomas from prestigious universities, always a good sign. He asked me questions about my health: all good, I told him. Fit as can be. Voice in perfect shape. You want a Turtle with martial arts skills, I can give you two of them.

After the visual inspection, he put on a rubber glove and said, "You're going to hate this."

I shuddered. "What end are you going for, pal?"

"Just come here," he said.

"I know I've had my head up my ass before," I said, "but if you've got to get to my throat that way, I'm in serious trouble."

A lame joke, but I was getting nervous. Shtick is one of my coping mechanisms. A little song, a little dance, a little seltzer down your pants, and chase those worries away.

He bent back my head, I opened my mouth, and he shoved his fingers down my throat. He spent ten or fifteen seconds poking around. He was down so deep it felt like he was somewhere between my mouth and my lungs. I had a world-class gag reflex. Fortunately I didn't have any Hungarian goulash that came up.

"I can't even feel a lump," he said, like it was my fault.

He pulled out and degloved and asked me questions about pain, weight loss, difficulty swallowing. I said no to all of the above. I really was feeling great—until now.

For the next examination, he went higher tech: a journey to the bottom of the earth with a laryngoscope. That's a fiber-optic camera used to get to deep dark places and see cool mucousy stuff. To numb me up for this photographic adventure, he squirted unpleasant stuff up my nose and it trickled down the back of my throat. It tasted vaguely of lemons. First came that weird tingling sensation of feeling like half my face was gone, like when I got smacked in the face with a hockey puck when I was a kid in Michigan.

Then he pushed the little camera up my nose, which didn't feel so little once it started plowing through my nostril.

The camera made a U-turn down my trachea to explore the back of my tongue and beyond. It was more uncomfortable than painful, like when you're drinking a Slurpee while driving and you slam on the brakes and the straw goes up your nose.

He had me position my head in such a way that I could see my vocal cords on a monitor. He then had me do a couple of different sounds— A, E, I, O, U. Then a couple of character voices. I was able to see how my vocal cords changed based on how I manipulated them, which was pretty fascinating.

He recorded a video, which I'd be able to get off the internet later. If nothing else, my windpipe might go viral.

The doctor informed me that he'd been the only ENT doc to have videotaped Mel Blanc's vocal cords while Mel was doing his famous voices. I had the same ENT guy who used to work on Bugs Bunny. "What's up, Doc?" indeed. How cool is that?

Looking at my vocal cords, he said, "Not a problem here. That's all great news—your vocal cords look perfect."

I asked him what the next step would be. He would prescribe antibiotics.

"If in fact it is an infection, this'll take care of it," he said. "I see nothing in your throat. Your voice sounds good. You're telling me you have no other symptoms. Let's give it ten days."

For the next week and a half, I was actually feeling pretty good. I touched the lump for the millionth time and told my wife, "You know, this is shrinking."

When I returned to the doctor, I told him the same thing.

"Nope," he said.

"What?"

"It's not getting smaller. Trust me."

He's got fifteen different plaques on his wall—who was I to disagree?

"Okay."

"Listen," he said, "I don't want to wait on this if it's what I think it is."

I didn't like the way he said *it*.

He asked me to go into one of the other examination rooms. He wanted to do a fine-needle aspiration to take a biopsy of the lump. He said normally he'd have another doctor do the procedure, but that would take two or three days to get an appointment.

"Would you mind if I just do it here?" he asked.

"Is it a big deal?" I asked.

"No, I might have to stick you a couple of times."

"We're here," I said, resigned. "Let's do it."

He gave me a little shot of lidocaine in the area of the lump and poked it half a dozen times with a very thin needle. It didn't hurt that much.

After he was done, I said, "What do you think?"

"Let's see," he said once again. "We'll wait for pathology and see what they say."

I asked him if worse came to worst, would it affect my voice? He explained that even if it was a tumor, it would be treatable, probably with chemotherapy and radiation.

The treatment would be a bitch, but I'd be cured and back on my feet, the recovery time uncertain but perhaps within months. Two years and I'd be myself again, more or less.

My mouth would take a beating, but since there was nothing showing on my vocal cords, there was a good chance I'd be able to talk. Whether I could still make funny voices or sing at a professional level, he couldn't say.

This was a Tuesday afternoon. As it happened, I had a gig that night at The Improv, the comedy club on Melrose Avenue in West Hollywood. My voice actor pals and I were doing *Talkin' Toons Live*. We do cartoon bits, song parodies, generally messing around for the audience. I record it for my podcast. I think we have as much fun as the crowd.

I ripped the Band-Aid off my neck and entered the club.

I don't remember much about the show except that it went great. I did a little stand-up for five or ten minutes and then I brought my guests onstage and we had a great time, as usual. Every now and then, I'd be taking a drink and I'd flash on what happened that day and go, *Holy shit, I might be really sick.* Then I'd return to performance mode.

It wasn't until I was making the long drive from the club in West Hollywood to my home northwest of Los Angeles that it began to sink in. My favorite satellite radio channel is the Sinatra channel. Frank's perfect phrasing both calmed me and sent my mind drifting, the way it does at night in the car with good music.

I remember thinking about my mother and how much I missed her. She was also a singer, and music had filled our home back in Michigan. In one respect I was glad she wasn't here anymore. She would have lost her mind over what was happening to one of her babies.

I thought about my dad, too. Our relationship was more complicated. I miss my mom every day. I miss my dad a few times a month. He'd totally get that.

I thought about the time I asked my business manager about insuring my voice, the way Cyd Charisse insured her legs. He didn't think it was worth it. There were only a couple of ways I'd collect. One was I would have to get injured in the throat so badly I couldn't talk, which seemed unlikely. I grew up playing hockey and remain a huge fan. There was a professional goalie who used to play for the Buffalo Sabres named Clint Malarchuk, whose throat got stepped on during a game. I watched a video of it on YouTube. It's just ghastly, because the other player's skate blade cut his jugular vein. My hockey days were over, so my neck was probably safe from skates, at least.

Another way was to get a disease of the throat.

As Sinatra did what Sinatra does best, I wondered what I would do if I lost my voice. Voice acting was my job, really the only long-term job I've ever had. I paid for everything—my kid's braces, toilet paper, and gasoline—with money I earned speaking and singing.

I thought about Yakko and what he'd say about somebody else doing his voice. "Who's the hack-o?" Carl Wheezer would ask, "What if the new guy doesn't have my signature lazy *l*? That's why chicks dig me." Raphael would roll with it. He's already been played by several other actors in other cartoon versions and in the big-screen films. "No big deal," he'd say. "When the movie guys did me, we worked with Megan Fox."

But it sure weighed on me, the options I might face. How else could I make a living? I'm a Ninja Turtle, for God's sake. If somebody said, "Here's the deal: we can save your life, but you're not going to sound the same," I really didn't know what the hell I would do.

Barista? Starbucks has great benefits, but I can only drink so much free coffee.

The joy I derive out of making myself and others laugh means everything to me. It goes to something that has been part of me as long as I can remember. Humor, music, creativity—it's all air to me. It feeds my soul and fuels my passion.

I couldn't imagine not having that. It's like a drug (and it doesn't leave any nasty track marks). To not be able to do those voices and not be able to feel that "drug" was terrifying.

Two days later, the doctor called.

"Hey, Rob, how are you feeling?"

"I don't know," I said. "How am I feeling?"

"Well," he said, "it's cancer."

CHAPTER TWO

Torpedoes in the Water

Let's get this out there up front. My father did not want me to become a professional actor.

"What the hell am I going to tell my friends?" he said.

I am the third Robert Paulsen, after the original, my grandfather, a Danish immigrant, and my American-born father, the junior. I felt like the entire weight of the immigrant experience pressed on my shoulders that day in the spring of 1975, when I told my parents that I was dropping out of the University of Michigan to pursue a career in showbiz.

"Look," I tried to explain, "I'm wasting your money and my time. I think I need to try show business."

My dad's remark hit me hard, like I'd been smacked to the ice by the biggest goon in the hockey rink. But I was determined. I didn't want to get my degree and jump into a job I didn't like just for the money. I wanted to sing and act.

My mom probably said something like, "Oh, Bob." I could tell she was torn. She wanted me to be happy but was obviously worried about me and trying to smooth things over with my father.

The irony is, I felt like they were the ones who had created this monster. I was probably two or three when I saw Elvis on TV. He was bumping and grinding to "Hound Dog." I couldn't take my eyes off him. I had to be the King of Rock and Roll. It was my parents who bought me a little guitar, one that you crank like a jack-in-the-box, and I would put on performances for friends and family.

"Ladies and gentlemen, introducing Robin Paulsen and his neckitar," my mom would announce, using the family nickname that set me apart from my father and grandfather.

I would shake my little hips and sing a song I made up called "You ain't nothing but an old ground hot dog."

It was my first musical parody. The adoring audience clapped, and that was all I needed. It was my first taste of performing, and I was hooked. As they say, the first one's free...

I'm from Michigan, which, if I hadn't written another two-hundred-plus pages, I'd suggest was all anybody needs to know about me. The state has a saying: "Pure Michigan." I tell people all the time that I'm Pure Michigan. Michigan gave me everything. I was born in 1956 in Detroit and moved around a lot: Livonia, Dearborn, Rochester, and finally high school in Grand Blanc, Michigan, just outside Flint, an hour by made-in-the-USA car north of Detroit.

It was a sweet little bedroom community for people who worked in Flint, in particular for Buick. In 1969, my mom and dad bought a lovely two-story colonial house with white aluminum siding in Grand Blanc. We were very middle-class, very vanilla. There was Mom and Dad and four kids and a collie named Rex (really). We couldn't have been any more white-bread, middle America if we had our own black-and-white sitcom. We were *The Donna Reed Show.*

I'm the oldest kid. My dad, Robert Paulsen Jr., was a salesman for Ryerson Steel of Detroit, driving around Michigan and Indiana and Ohio selling steel. My mom was a full-time housewife with a capital *F* and, for my money, one of the most remarkable women in the world... just like your mother.

My mother, a really wonderful singer, was in the Miss Detroit competition in the '40s, and her talent was singing. My father could sing, too. They both had a deep love of Broadway musical theater. The soundtracks from *The Music Man*, *My Fair Lady*, and *West Side Story* streamed out of the hi-fi console.

I can't remember a time when music wasn't a part of my life. My brother and sisters—Mike, Lori, and Shelley—all became pretty damn good singers, too. They favored choir. I loved rock and roll. At about age eleven, I got a drum set from my folks, and I'd go down in the basement and beat the Christ out it.

As I grew older, my parents were very clear: I could listen to as much Beatles and Dave Clark Five and Led Zeppelin as I wanted, as long as I also listened to Mahler and Rachmaninoff, some Johnny Mercer and Jule Styne, and the Gershwins. I developed a deep appreciation for all kinds of music and understood how all these musicians were inspired by each other. My Danish immigrant grandparents on my father's side loved Denmark's own Victor Borge. We sat around and watched him on *The Tonight Show*, and even at ten years old I knew he was really special. He'd play a melody that sounded familiar but you couldn't quite place it. Then he would turn the sheet music right side up and it was the "William Tell Overture." Genius.

At Grand Blanc High School I was a good, not great, student, prone to distraction and goofing around in class. I was already making funny voices. Who knew that I would one day make my living doing what got me in trouble in home room? My report cards reflected this: *Rob's a nice boy, very funny, very clever, does not apply himself. Not genius.*

As a kid growing up in the northern Midwest, Gordie Howe was my hero, though I never dreamed that one day I'd meet the Red Wings legend at a charity event. I was assistant captain, varsity three years, a swift and agile skater on the left wing, and I entertained dreams of becoming a professional until a big kid from Manitoba knocked me on my ass and turned my nose sideways.

But even as I kept one foot (skate?) in sports, music became my passion. I was lucky to have teachers who understood my urge to perform and encouraged me. A gifted teacher named Caroline Mawby insisted I learn to read music and take a theory class, and she got me into choir, where I was a first tenor.

I also hung around with a group of guys who had long hair and were shy and awkward and obsessed with music. People called them freaks. They weren't into drugs or anything; they didn't drink, didn't smoke, never hit a reefer. But they embraced their reputation and created a band called LS Phreaque, making me lead singer.

The guys were amazing musicians. We learned the usual covers for the 1970s: Led Zeppelin, The Who, the Stones. The first time I hit the stage with them, it was a revelation. I felt at home. It made sense in a way—for as long as I can remember, for better or worse, I have craved attention. But only under certain circumstances. If I were called on in class to describe the Pythagorean theorem, I would crumble. Put me among friends and let me try to make them laugh, I would light up.

The same applied to singing. Audience members have always felt like my friends. I suspect that's because I feel like I'm safe onstage. I'm the person who decides what comes out of my mouth, even if it's someone else's lyrics. I put my spin on the song, curling a note here and there to make it my own. And in the context of the band, I wasn't up there by myself. I had the support of the other guys around me. We weren't the Rob Paulsen Experience. We were a group, like a hockey team.

The first few times our band played, it was for only our friends, essentially. The feedback was quick and positive, and I found a level of acceptance among my peers that I hadn't seen in other areas of my life. Had we really sucked, I don't know how I would have turned out. But we were good. And when we weren't, I figured out that self-effacing humor solves almost every problem. If I flubbed a lyric, I'd say, "Good thing I look hot in tight jeans, because I can't remember a word."

As we began to play for people who didn't know us personally, I realized I could still suss out the crowd, still sense what to do and when. I had a fearlessness that came from youth and from knowing I had found my place in the world. I certainly had nerves before each gig, but I was never *nervous*. It was more the excitement I'd get from not wanting to wait another second to get out there and show them what I could do. Our principal was a great guy who let us play at school assemblies. We thought we were the coolest—total rebels when we played "Smokin' in the Boys Room."

. While I was always encouraged in music, I had my share of talks with my father, even back then. "How come you know every lyric to every song but you stink in math?" The subtext, usually unspoken, sometimes not, was that music mattered, but only to a point. That point ended when music threatened to conflict with schoolwork or finding a solid job. It was an attitude that grated on me.

I want to be clear: I really loved my parents. To this day, I constantly ask myself if my parents would approve of my behavior. But when I was onstage, I was trying to find my own way, on my own terms, as a performer, as Rob. Onstage, my parents couldn't touch me. Onstage, I was in control.

It wasn't long before I realized I was a better performer than hockey player. I knew where I was going. The question was how to get there.

Our band recorded a single at the house of one of my friends, Bob Lamb. His dad was a local celebrity with a radio program he broadcast from his basement called the *Buick Factory Whistle Show*. Mr. Lamb's studio had world-class recording equipment, and that's where we cut our first and only original single. It was pretty awful, and we never wrote another, but we were a tight cover band.

Our senior year we won a battle of the bands, determined by audience applause, and as a prize got to open for Bob Seger. This was about 1974, and our little band played in Davisburg, an outdoor amphitheater with about three thousand people, by far our biggest crowd. Of course the audience was there to see Bob Seger, and they were giving us a hard time. We got a smattering of boos and a lot of hostile restlessness. Nobody threw anything (that would happen later). I was eighteen or nineteen, standing up there, disconcerted and overwhelmed.

As the crowd grew surly, something happened I'll never forget. Bob Seger came out and took the mic from me. He admonished the crowd. "Look, these guys have earned the right to be here," he said. "I'll be out here when it's time; otherwise, these guys deserve your respect."

They immediately embraced us. I don't know Bob; I know some of his people. I sure would love to tell him one day what an example that was to me as a young person of how to handle celebrity and be a professional. Pure Michigan. Pure class.

I bumbled through school during that time in my life, tired from coming home late after rehearsing with my band or playing a prom gig for fifty bucks or, in winter, getting up at 5:30 a.m. for hockey practice. But I managed to do well enough that, after graduating in 1974, I got into the University of Michigan–Flint.

We were all big Wolverines fans, and the fact that my parents' oldest child got accepted to school made their dreams come true. I took general studies with vague designs on being, of all things, a dentist, probably because of my hockey experience. I'd seen so many busted teeth that I thought dentistry wasn't a bad way to make a living.

It didn't take me long to realize that I was not in my element. I wasn't so good at going to class, because I was listening to music, hanging out with buddies, playing in a band. All I wanted was free time to be creative and musical and comedic with like-minded people. Then, one day, my high school friend Chuck Neighbors called me. He had gone to LA and joined a small itinerant theater company. It was a faith-based group that traveled around the country doing little plays and musical skits to spread the word.

Nobody ever accused the Paulsens of Grand Blanc of being overly religious, or even theologically consistent. I was baptized in the Eastern Orthodox Church. My father was Lutheran. If we went to church, it was because somebody got married or died, and then we usually went to a Presbyterian church.

"Even if you're not religious, you'll dig this," my friend insisted. The troupe performed in churches and before groups like the Salvation Army—even in prisons. I would get my basic expenses covered and receive a small stipend. More importantly, I would get to perform professionally. And the skits included singing parts.

The offer intrigued me, though I knew my parents would object. I considered transferring to the American Academy of Dramatic Arts, an acting school in Los Angeles where I could also earn a bachelor's degree. This would serve as a compromise, but at the time I worried about my acting chops. The school required an audition. I was a singer, not an actor, and I didn't think I could hack it.

As I broke the news to my parents about leaving college, I knew they would be unhappy, but my father's reaction stuck in my craw. By all accounts I was a pretty good kid, and I tried to live up, as best I could, to his military standards. I kept my hair short even though I sang in a rock band. I was the assistant captain of the hockey team, a four-year letterman. I wasn't a star pupil, but I got good enough grades to land me at UM–Flint. I did my chores, and I stayed out of trouble. I thought I had earned my parents' trust.

Music had become my passion, and I was good at it, but my dad refused to recognize this. He demeaned my music and therefore demeaned me. That he would throw his disappointment in my face broke my heart. I wanted to tell him, "Sure, you went to my hockey games, and I'm glad you did, but that was because hockey interested you. You never saw me onstage. You never saw me shine. I would have made you proud. But it didn't interest you."

I wanted to tell him a lot of things.

Many years later, having raised my own Paulsen boy to adulthood, I came to understand his point of view. My parents were born in the late '20s, children of the Depression. Their parents had come through Ellis Island so that their children and grandchildren could thrive and succeed and experience the American dream. The fact that I was dropping out of college probably made him feel like *he* was the failure, not me.

But my younger self didn't understand that yet. My younger self swallowed hard and resolved that one day I would show him.

Not the worst reaction by young Rob, all things considered. America in the 1970s offered a lot of dark and dangerous roads for a rebellious white kid from the Midwest: drugs, cults, disco. I was joining a Christian-based arts organization, not the Symbionese Liberation Army. But my resolve also meant I sidestepped a difficult conversation with my father, one that would have required both of us to summon more honesty than either of us was perhaps capable of at the time.

For as long as I can remember, this had been a constant between us—the sweep-the-tough-stuff-under-the-rug approach—and my mother was often a conspirator. When I was in junior high school, I got a D in a class. Terrified of what my dad would say, I used a fine-tipped pen to change that D into a B. I finally fessed up to my mom, begging her not to tell my dad. She went along with it, and this set a precedent for evasion and improvisation that would serve me well as a performer, but also more than once bite me in the ass as a person.

To their credit, my parents didn't try to stop me from trying to make a living in show business. But they didn't make it easy, either. They said they loved me, that I would always be their son, but that they thought I was making a big mistake. They also made clear that the money that followed me to college wouldn't follow me to Los Angeles.

With a gulp, I said, "I know."

A few days later, Chuck called about the theater group. "Hey, man, they're really gearing up," he said. "You need to be out there now."

I had to make a decision. A plane ticket was waiting for me. It was a Saturday, and my parents weren't around. My dad loved to sail, and

19

he and my mom were with friends on a forty-footer on Lake Huron. There was no ship-to-shore radio, no cell phones in those days.

Unsure what to do, I called my grandfather.

Robert Paulsen Sr. was raised in a small, cold Danish town called Faaborg in the Baltic. He was a learned person, a mechanical engineer, and when he got to the US he first worked in tool and die shops. This was during World War I, and he was always careful not to say too much because his Danish sounded like German, and he was afraid of getting the shit beat out of him.

During World War II, he was hired by the US government to make the glass ocular components of bomb sights in his basement shop. He had security clearances, and while he was not a military guy, he had a loaded gun, just in case.

He also had a wonderfully dry sense of humor. One night my family was over at his house when my grandfather came through the door.

"What did the doctor say, Bob?" asked my grandmother, who was named Matilda Henrietta, but everyone called her Tilly.

"Apparently, I have cancer," he said. "What's for dinner?"

I'm sure there was one of those long, awkward silences as we watched my grandfather calmly go about his business.

I was probably about sixteen. I couldn't figure out if he was incredibly brave or extremely weird. He was in his seventies at the time and, although nobody spoke about it—cancer was a dirty word in those days—I think it was probably prostate cancer. He beat the disease and lived well into his eighties.

As I got older, I came to have great respect for my grandfather. And when I had to make a snap decision about leaving for Los Angeles and couldn't contact my parents, I reached out to him.

"I understand you wanting to follow your dream," he told me. "I also understand it not being popular with your parents."

He recalled that he was about my age when he decided to leave Denmark, with plans of hopping on a ship from Copenhagen to Halifax and entering the United States near Niagara Falls. The *Lusitania* had recently been sunk, and the ocean waters were dangerous.

"People told me, 'Robert, you cannot go across the North Atlantic right now because there are torpedoes in the water,'" my grandfather said. "People will always tell you that there are torpedoes in the water."

It was such a poetic way of saying it, one of the best lessons. Damning the torpedoes, he did come to the United States, and he said he was a better man for it—otherwise he'd never have the joy of speaking to his grandchild now. He said he would talk to my parents when they got back. I scribbled a note on the back of a grocery receipt telling my parents that I was flying to Los Angeles and would call them when I arrived.

It was June of 1975. I got on my first ever big-time plane flight, Detroit Metro to LAX, and headed to the land of The Doors and *Happy Days*.

After I landed and made my way over the Sepulveda Pass into the San Fernando Valley, I was overwhelmed and disoriented. There were palm trees and all these beautiful cars that had no rust on them. For those accustomed to sunnier climates, this wouldn't have been a novelty. But in Michigan, the highway department sprinkled salt on the roads to melt the snow, and the salt wreaked havoc on bumpers and undercarriages alike.

I called my house from a pay phone.

"Where are you?" my mother asked.

"I'm in Hollywood. I'm where I told you I would be."

"No, *where* are you?"

"St. James Presbyterian Church," I said. "In Reseda."

Okay, not exactly Hollywood. Reseda's not even Encino. But I had arrived.

The Covenant Players were formed by Charles Tanner, a TV writer who had become a born-again Christian. He decided that he would use his talents to become a witness for Christianity. It was a faith-based group, but it was wide-open. I made friends who were Christian. I made friends who were Jewish, which wasn't a religion I'd encountered in my hometown. I heard the term *Wiccan* for the first time. I thought the girl was saying *wicker*. She said, "No, my mom's a witch."

I was hooked up with four or five other people who had a group leader. We squeezed into an Econoline van, where I gagged on cigarette smoke, because everybody smoked in those days, and traveled the country doing prebooked shows.

The first tour covered Northern California. We stayed in churches, sleeping on floors and on couches. These were people I hadn't known a few weeks earlier, and now I was on the road with them. We were spreading the gospel via our theatrical plays—short, two-person plays based on moral themes. For example, one character would amble onto stage, minding his own business, maybe smoking a cigarette because you could do that in the theater in those days, and he'd see the second character, a woman, high atop a fifty-foot skyscraper, ready to jump to her death. Of course, she was only on a folding chair, but with good enough acting we could make it seem real. Cigarette guy, often me, would then wonder aloud just what in God's name he should do, God being the important element.

It was smart writing by Mr. Tanner. We would end the scene and then open it up for a discussion with the audience. What do we do when we encounter somebody in distress? Do we just have a smoke and move on? Do we talk to them? What do we say?

I would realize later that these performances taught me so much more about how acting, music, and laughter could be tools. The Covenant Players would be the superstructure for what, to this day, drives me to perform—the chance to affect people on a much deeper level.

Although the plays were overtly Christianity based, we were invited to perform for a variety of faiths. I got to meet rabbis who would host us. We performed in mosques. I met conservative Christians who weren't allowed to dance and sing. I met Catholic priests drinking wine and telling me the dirtiest jokes. Many of these folks were working in the trenches, with the poorest of the poor, in soup kitchens and homeless shelters.

Once, we got invited by the chaplain at San Quentin State Prison to come in and spend a day doing scenes for a select group of inmates. When you're working around people who are saying, "Hey, motherfucker," and "Come here and I'll cut your throat," you tend to learn a lot about concentration and stagecraft.

It was this practical experience I craved: how to pick up cues, what to do when you see that blank stare from another actor that means they've forgotten their line. I learned how to deal with being thrown into the water in the deep end. I learned how to take an emotional punch when I didn't have a particularly good performance.

Our little troupe of five squeezed into a van and rode for hours a day, gagging on everyone else's cigarette smoke, getting on each other's nerves. Homesickness, petty disputes, ego trips—it all came into play. Then at night we had to put it aside so we could go onstage and completely concentrate, learning how to put all of our trust into that colleague we were ready to strangle two hours earlier.

We had to become professionals, whether we felt like it or not, because it was all about the audience. Whether they paid in money or in their time, we had to do something that was worthy of their coming to see us.

As much as I was getting out of this experience, my dad never really did understand why I joined Covenant Players. We did a tour of the eastern part of the United States, and along the way the troupe met my parents.

"This is your show business?" my dad said.

"It's experience," I said.

"What the hell's this guy's experience," he said of the leader, "being forty years old in a bus?"

I didn't even try to explain it.

As my one-year commitment neared an end, the home office in Reseda suggested that I stay on as a group leader. I was flattered, and I considered it for a while. The group gave me the chance to be in front of people, making them think and laugh and cry. The second half of the tour even included music, and every night I could perform religious pop songs accompanied by a cassette player.

But in the end, I told them I appreciated the offer but I was going to move on. It was a pleasant parting, bittersweet for maybe both of us. I had wanted to stay in Los Angeles and try other forms of acting, but I was at the mercy of my circumstances. That is to say, I had no money, no car, no apartment. I had been living out of a van for a year. I needed someplace safe and cheap where I could get my shit together and figure out how to make it work in LA.

In the summer of 1976, I moved back home. My parents were welcoming, but they had a message: it's nice to have you here, glad you had a wonderful experience with the Covenant Players, now get a real job.

After spending a year and change enjoying the creative process and having romantic flings and entertaining prisoners and performing before countless numbers of interesting people I never would have met otherwise, I was back in Michigan, unemployed. I found work as a short-order cook at Perkins pancake house in Grand Blanc while my parents started in on me about returning to school now that I'd gotten this acting thing out of my system. But I was smitten. I had gotten to sing. I had gotten to be a soloist. It hadn't been glamorous, but it felt like that was what I was here to do.

Pinocchio, I hear you, man: hi-diddle-dee-dee, an actor's life for me.

Just as my parents were pushing me to go to junior college in the fall to prepare to transfer back to the University of Michigan, some of my old friends from LS Phreaque told me about a rock band called Sass, based in Lake Fenton, Michigan, that was looking for a singer. I thought anything was better than making eggs and pancakes.

I hopped in my mom's white Chevy Monte Carlo and headed twelve miles down Fenton Road to the Lake Fenton Country Club, where Sass had a standing gig in the restaurant/bar next to the golf course. It was a warm evening, and I had on my jeans and a T-shirt as I walked into the lounge, which housed a small stage, maybe eight by ten feet. I arrived on a Saturday night, and the house was going to be packed. That was part of the deal. They wanted me to rehearse a couple of songs then perform in front of their crowd on their busiest night. For some people, this might sound terrifying. I was like: *bring it.*

By day, the restaurant served as a beer and cocktail lounge for the golfers, but at night it was all nightclub. I took the stage in my cowboy boots; I was into cowboy boots in those days. I breathed in. The joint smelled of stale beer, cigarette smoke, and vomit, an aroma that became as familiar to me as Mom's apple pie and Grandma's fried chicken—the cologne of my life. I still miss it.

We played the three songs we had rehearsed, an eclectic set so the guys could test my range. The first two were "This Masquerade" by Leon Russell and George Benson, then "Rikki Don't Lose that Number" by Steely Dan. We closed out the set with "Won't Get Fooled Again" by The Who. This was not classic rock back then; that song was still a recent hit.

The song has two big moments, those seminal Roger Daltrey screams, the biggest one coming after a long Hammond-B3-organ-through-Leslie-speaker interlude, which the keyboardist, Denis Ikeler, played perfectly. It's the same scream that has opened one of those *CSI* TV shows for years. And during rehearsal, I couldn't get it right. I nailed the vocals but muffed the timing. The bass player, Jack Regis, was supposed to set me up—one, two, three, four—followed by me going "AAAAAAAHHHHHHHH," before the song's famous wind-mill power chords roared. Only I couldn't hear the bass player and kept coming in late or early, which can be a huge problem when you're screeching at the top of your lungs.

We got through the first two songs of the gig easily. Then we started playing "Won't Get Fooled Again." For such a small stage, the band brought big effects, including killer lights and their own smoke machine (it was a fifty-five-gallon drum with hot water in it; at the appointed moment, their manager would drop in dry ice and smoke would billow out, as it was doing now, during that long keyboard section).

As my big moment approached, I realized I now couldn't hear *or* see. But if I didn't nail this scream, it was back to soul-crushing pan-cake flipping.

Through the fog, I could just make out Regis. He had said, "Watch me like a hawk." The rest of the band, including guitarist Dennis Briggs and drummer John Hill, were lost in the haze. As Ikeler ended the solo, Regis mouthed, "One, two, three—" On *four* I dug deep into my soul and screamed my lungs out. I think I triggered cave-ins on two sand traps on the back nine.

I don't remember what the audience did. It didn't matter. I could see it in the guys' faces. We took a break, shook hands, and they said, "Let's do this." The next day, I gave my notice at Perkins.

This was the summer of 1976. Singing for Sass was a grind in the best possible way, six nights a week, 8:00 p.m. to 2:00 a.m., with only Mondays off. We did five sets a night with twenty-minute breaks. In the beginning there weren't too many crowds on a Tuesday night in Midland or a Thursday night in Saginaw. But word got around that these guys were good, and we started to build an audience. We went from being a quaint little bar band to a really excellent cover band with our own following.

It was trial by fire, like the Covenant Players, but even more intense. I learned what to do if I screwed up onstage or the equipment broke down, both of which happened all the time and always at the worst possible times. Mostly, I learned what it takes to be a professional performer: the willingness to understand that you've got room to improve, that you don't know it all, that you need to rise to the level of those around you.

I also learned what happens when a loud drunk guy requests a song but you don't play it because you don't know it (he threw a shot glass at my head). And I learned what happens when you get too friendly with a girl who apparently also appealed to a biker guy (he went into the parking lot and smashed my car windshield; I drove home in Michigan in November with the arctic air hitting me in the face).

The guys in Sass gave me the confidence to get better. As a lead singer, I thought of myself as a poor man's Robert Plant—actually, a broke man's Robert Plant. I didn't have the gobs of hair or the private jet, but I could hit the notes when I had to. As a high tenor, I sang more like Kenny Loggins, with a lighter voice, but one I could stretch. The guys helped me with close harmonies and other nuances of the music. Before Sass, I had gotten by on instinct; they turned me from a singer into a musician.

I gained so much confidence that I started thinking beyond the band. The turning point came one night when we were playing at our home club, Mr. G's, which was full every night. We played everything: an eclectic lineup of rock, blues, pop, and standards. Sass had developed a following by this point. One of our diehard fans who followed us everywhere was a man named Mickey. He was probably a budding alcoholic but deeply committed to all things Sass. We were doing a Zeppelin tune, and when the song ended, Mickey was still screaming at the top of his lungs with a Heineken in each hand, completely tanked.

"Hey, Rob," he said, coming up to me at a break.

"Hey, Mickey, what's up?" I said.

"You're the best band in Flint," he said.

It was one of those moments where the little angel on my shoulder said, "Hey, man, he's right. You are the best band in Flint, especially since Grand Funk Railroad became real rock 'n' roll stars and don't live here anymore." This was as good as it was going to get.

I was almost twenty-two. I had already been kicking around the idea that we'd all go out to LA together. I thought we had a chance of making it big. But the band was booked a year in advance, and they weren't interested. A couple of the guys were married and very comfortable in the gig.

Michigan was fine with them. It just wasn't fine with me.

Not long after that, I told them they better start looking for a new singer. Although I didn't have a job lined up, I decided to go for this second round in LA. Little did I know there were things afoot that would shape my future dramatically, things happening that I didn't or couldn't understand, things involving grease, potatoes, onions, and salt.

Actually, they were not things at all.

They were Frings. And they would rock my world.

CHAPTER THREE

My First Hollywood Fring

My mother was standing on the porch of our little home in her chenille bathrobe, just like in the movies, her oldest child heading back to Hollywood to be in the movin' pitcher bidness.

I had a sense, this time, that I wouldn't be coming back as I had before. I left my hockey stuff at home. And I never did return to Michigan for more than short visits. The longest was maybe two weeks when I got married.

In June of '78, I drove out to LA with my buddy Bob Lamb. He also had been in LA before. We both wanted to be close to the ocean, so we decided to check out the South Bay, somewhere in Redondo, Hermosa, Manhattan Beach, or Torrance. We arrived in mid-June. The first two nights we stayed in Hermosa Beach in a motel called the Sand Dollar or the Sand Piper or the Sand Castle; sand was involved, I remember that much. It was a notch below Motel 6, but the sheets seemed clean enough and, anyway, we were in California. On the third day of apartment hunting, we found a vacancy sign outside the Esplanade Village Apartments, across the street from the beach in Redondo Beach. The apartment managers, Betty and Leonard Peterson, couldn't have been nicer. They knew right away we had no jobs but took a chance on us. I had $1,300 in cash that I had saved up for my trip to LA. By the time we paid our first and last month's rent, I was pretty much broke. They gave us the apartment anyway.

Although I didn't have a job lined up, I knew the lay of the land. I was not that much older, but a lot wiser. I knew that I could handle disappointment. I knew what it took to get back on my feet. I knew that the odds were not in my favor. I knew I needed a lot of luck. But I was ready to suck it up and get odd jobs and put myself in a position where I could get lucky.

The first time it was overwhelming. Now it was just whelming.

God bless Betty and Leonard. Knowing my employment situation, they helped the kid out, hiring me as their handyman. I cleaned the units and fixed the toilets and sinks and did minor electrical work. I was able to make rent, and I had time to go about trying to become a star.

I pored through *Drama-Logue* and *Backstage* and other magazines and auditioned for everything I could find. A few weeks after getting to LA, in August of '78, I landed a gig on a cable show called *Shake a Leg*. I say cable; this was local access. We shot it in a little studio in Santa Monica. It was nonunion. I was singing and dancing and doing wacky skits with a young lady whose name I don't remember (I want to say Mandy?). The gig lasted only weeks, and the show was probably all a tax write-off for somebody. To this day I've never actually seen it. If anybody out there has a YouTube video, let me know!

But it became an important stepping stone. The wardrobe lady put me in touch with an agent named Debbie Dozier. Debbie's father was Bill Dozier, who executive produced the original *Batman* TV show, and her mother was the legendary actress Joan Fontaine. I remember telling my mother that I knew Joan Fontaine's daughter. My mom was very impressed.

Debbie didn't sign me, but she suggested I reach out to a commercial agent named Dick Barth, one of the three partners of the agency Sutton, Barth & Vennari. In late 1978, I started writing Dick letters and calling him, because that's what Debbie Dozier said I should do. That was in the day before email, so all the notes were typed and sent by mail.

I finally reached Dick on the phone. He said he couldn't sign me at the time but encouraged me to keep in touch. Which I did, with probably more enthusiasm than he appreciated. I showered him with letters and head shots and continued to bug him by phone for months while I auditioned for showcases and plays and did pro bono singing on demo tapes for musician friends.

It turned out my timing was excellent. Sutton, Barth & Vennari was brand-new, the partners having spun off from another agency, and they were seeking a lot of actors to build their stable of clients. In May of 1979, after months of me pestering him, Dick said, "Okay, come into the office."

They were on Beverly Boulevard and Sweetzer in West Holly-wood, Suite 310. I went upstairs and read for Dick. He was at his desk, watching me. Dick was a tall, handsome guy and all business—not unpleasant, but not overly friendly. I'd later find out that he was active in the National Audubon Society and a dedicated bird-watcher. If I was a species that interested him, you'd never have known it from his blank expression.

I don't remember what the copy was, just typical stuff for a TV commercial appropriate for a boy child from Michigan. When I fin-ished reading, Dick simply shook my hand and said, "Go down the hall and the secretary will have contracts for you. Welcome aboard."

Just like that, after nearly a year of banging on doors in Hollywood, they let me in. I got in my car, tossed my freshly signed contracts on the seat, and thought of all those actors on award shows saying, "I want to thank my agent." Now I was one of those actors. *Maybe I should work on my acceptance speech.*

I stopped along the way to get fancy new head shots taken. Back then, I would describe myself as the all-American, average-looking Caucasian boy. I looked younger than my age. I had kind of a mullet, a reflection not only of the times, but of my hockey background. A lot of hockey players favored the business-in-the-front, party-in-the-back look.

I don't think I was a particularly good-looking kid. I was five ten, a buck sixty-five, in good shape, but no six-pack abs. I was very vanilla. I'd never get the hunky roles, but I had a look that many producers wanted at the time. That, and my vanilla voice—lower tenor register, vaguely somewhere middle-America sounding—gave me great tools to work with in the late '70s.

Average was the place to be.

When I got home, there was a message on the answering machine. "It's Dick Barth," he said. His voice had a touch of surprise that worried me for a second. "Nice meeting you today. Uh, we have an audition for you. Your call time is ten o'clock in the morning. Wear a nice shirt and take your head shot and résumé."

He rattled off the address and added, "It's for Jack in the Box."

Growing up in Grand Blanc, we had Bob's Big Boy and McDonald's and Burger King. But I had never had the pleasure of driving up to a clown and placing my order for Jumbo Jacks and deep-fried tacos.

I had seen Jack in the Boxes around LA, and I may have picked up a burger—I honestly don't remember. I certainly wasn't privy to Jack's latest marketing campaign and had no idea what Jack wanted from me as I arrived at the casting office on La Brea in Hollywood.

I would come to see countless casting offices like this over the years, a nothing-looking building off a boulevard with offices lit by fluorescent bulbs. Hollywood only looks glamorous from the outside. This is where the real business is done.

As I awaited my turn to read, I felt confident. I already had a pretty good idea how to audition on camera, having done songs and dances for that goofy *Shake a Leg* show. I had been on live stages for the Covenant Players, performed in nightclubs all over Michigan for Sass, and gotten booed by Bob Seger fans.

The casting agency staff summoned me into a little room, where I stood in front of a firing squad of ad agency people and Jack in the Box representatives. I had a little bit of copy to memorize; there was no teleprompter.

Then off I went, doing my thing, playing the all-American boy, happy as shit to be eating Jack in the Box. They said thank you very much, and I went back to the Esplanade Village Apartments.

Later that afternoon I got a call from Dick Barth.

"You booked that Jack in the Box commercial," he said. "Congratulations."

He again seemed a little surprised. I thought it was the most natural thing in the world, getting a TV commercial on one of my first auditions within hours of getting signed by an agency. That's how I thought Hollywood always worked. Still, I didn't have a clue what I was supposed to do next for Jack in the Box. Dick explained there would be a wardrobe fitting the next day and they would shoot the day after that.

I hung up and said, "Holy. Shit."

Two days later, I was on location at an actual Jack in the Box somewhere in Hollywood, the restaurant having been shut down for the commercial. The place was full of expensive-looking lights and cameras and microphones and crew people who all seemed to know what they were doing, unlike me.

They sent me off to get my wardrobe, and I was transformed into a Jack in the Box counter guy, down to the white dress shirt, tie, paper hat, and name tag. "Larry," I think it said, or maybe "Stanley."

I memorized my (very few) lines and assumed my position behind the counter. Behind the big Panaflex camera sat the director, the wonderful Hobby Morrison, a veteran of commercials who had done it all and seen it all.

He said, "Action."

With my big Michigan grin, I said, "Have a Fring!"

Few people may remember Jack's would-be great innovation in fast casual dining. Frings—one-half fries, one-half onion rings—will never be studied in business schools and culinary institutes for the simple reason that nobody wanted to buy them. It seemed you were either in the fries camp or the rings camp; to combine them was unnatural, in the fast-food sense.

This would come to my attention later. At the time, I was doing my best to impress upon the director and the suits on set my unmitigated, heartfelt joy at everything Fringy.

Which is why it was so disconcerting that after every take the people from the ad agency would whisper to Morrison, who would nod and then tell me to do another take. Sometimes they'd whisper to him while I was delivering the lines, and again he'd tell me to do it again.

It began to weigh on me. When I came out to LA, I had dreams of working a sweeping David Lean epic on location for six months in Morocco. How could I fuck up a Jack in the Box commercial?

After about twelve takes of the same line, one of the ad agency women said, "Hang on, just a second, stop everything."

I figured I would be fired on the spot. Instead she came up to me and adjusted the employee name tag on my shirt. She backed up, and looked at it, and said, "Great, now let's go."

Problem solved—we shot it again and everybody was satisfied.

Later, Hobby told me, "Rob, we got this on the first take. I work with these people all the time. If they ask you to stand on your head and pick your nose, just do it. The longer we're here, the more money we make."

Hobby put me at ease and taught me a terrific lesson: I didn't take it personally. I went about my business as a professional.

Decades later, when I became a voice director on the latest incarnation of the Ninja Turtles franchise, I emulated Hobby's style. Actors tend toward insecurity and self-involvement under the best of circumstances. Younger ones can be terrified that if they do a single thing wrong they'll never work in this town again.

Hobby taught me how important it was to understand that it's not always about the actor. When I'm directing in a room with four writers, and each one has an idea of how a line should be delivered, it can be a dozen takes before we're done. By then the actor is a wreck, thinking they've messed up. That's when I take them aside, remind them to keep breathing, and tell them we nailed it the first time. The rest was just gravy.

I wrapped up the Jack in the Box shoot and returned to the Esplanade apartments as the Petersons' handyman. I didn't mind. It was a great job because it gave me the flexibility to go out on auditions, which began to roll in.

For the next few weeks, I continued reading for casting agents until one day I was summoned to an apartment unit where an old woman had something stuck in her drain. As she watched *The Price Is Right*, I squeezed under the kitchen sink, removed the sink trap, retrieved an old sponge, blew out the trap, and put it back together.

I was still under the counter, my ass up in the air, when this sweet old lady said something I'll never forget: "Oh my goodness, you look just like the guy in the Jack in the Box commercial."

CHAPTER FOUR

Where's the Cum Shot?

That fast food clown opened a lot of doors. After the Jack in the Box commercial, my name got around town, and casting directors called me in to read for commercials for Buick, Ford, Levi's, Bullock's and The Broadway department stores, Coke and Pepsi, Baskin-Robbins. I wasn't picky. The only brands off-limits to me were other fast-food chains like McDonald's and Wendy's. My Jack in the Box contract had a no-compete clause. For the next thirteen weeks I was Jack's man, and any dreams of being the next Hamburglar would have to wait.

I ended up doing probably twenty-five or thirty TV commercials over the following years. I had no illusions about my talent. It was mostly about my bland looks and accessible personality. I was a twenty-three-year-old kid with this natural effervescence, an innocence that is appealing in the context of a commercial for bread or Clorox. I was the boy next door to the little girl who says, "Allen, I can help you get that gravy stain out."

Along with helping me get auditions and other commercials, the Jack in the Box gig solved the old catch-22 for actors. It's difficult to get an acting job if you aren't a member of the union, the Screen Actors Guild, but you can't get a SAG card unless you do a SAG job.

Jack in the Box secured a waiver from SAG to hire me under the auspices of the union, with the understanding I'd get my SAG card upon completion of the shoot.

Jack also got me into the other big union. An agent at the firm who handled voice actors called me asking if I had my AFTRA card. Jack in the Box wanted me to do radio commercials for the Frings. In those days, it was the medium that dictated the union that covered you. If it was a film gig, on camera, or an animated film show, it was a SAG project. If it was a videotape show like a soap opera, or radio or music, it was under the American Federation of Television and Radio Artists. (The two unions have since merged).

I did the voice-over work, and now I was also an AFTRA actor. At the time, I was working for the union minimum. SAG scale was about $500 for a TV commercial, and AFTRA scale was $250 for a radio spot, with residuals depending on how often the ads aired and in how many markets. So nearly everything I made from Jack went to the unions in the form of dues, which was fine with me, because I was in the same union as Robert Redford. Even though I was still cleaning apartments, I could proudly call myself a working Hollywood actor, and I was on my way toward someday getting health insurance under the union.

One day I went to the mailbox and got a pleasant surprise. Jack in the Box had sent me my first residuals check for commercials playing around the country. It was like Christmas. Even after my agents took their 10 percent, I felt like I was sitting in high cotton.

And just like that, I was seduced by fame and money.

Now, this is the part in most celebrity memoirs where my life would devolve into a world of Hollywood excess. I suppose that could have happened to me if a) I were an actual celebrity; and b) that check was for more than $2,000. But that check still had a negative effect on me.

When I went to auditions, I was nervous. Instead of concentrating on letting them see my talent, I was thinking: Don't blow this line. Cash is at stake.

I looked around, and friends were booking pilots. Some of those pilots were going to series. Now you're talking serious money, like $15,000 a week. I was a sports car geek and still am, and one of my goals was to have my own Porsche 911. I would go to the dealership in Hermosa Beach and talk to the mechanics, telling them that one day I was going to get me one of those German sports cars. Then a guy in my acting class showed up with a brand-new Porsche because he had just booked a series, and I was doubly determined.

It ended up tainting my performances at auditions. The innocence and excitement and effervescence that I would bring to my reads were dulled. There was a whiff of desperation.

And professional casting people, especially once they get to know you, can smell desperation instantly.

The callbacks became less frequent, and I would get messages on my machine from casting agents like, "Hey, Robbie, you just didn't hit on this one. Maybe next time."

"Next time" can mean "never" in Hollywood. Then if I got a callback, I'd be even more desperate: audition, followed by the sound of a phone not ringing. I'd call my agent and he'd say, "They decided to go with somebody else."

I came to realize that the margin of error in Hollywood was razor thin. These auditions had two hundred guys who looked exactly like me. I was still delivering good reads. But that little tiny something, that sparkle or whatever the hell it was, had gone away, replaced by a scared little guy thinking, *I need this job.*

This fixation on money was the antithesis of what it was that got me out to LA in the first place: that pure desire to perform that had me doing that dumb cable show and sending out those letters and banging on those doors to get an agent. My lack of work was a stark, immediate reminder that you can't get too full of yourself. You may get to live the dream for a couple of hours, with your own dressing room trailer and free food and a little plaque with your name on the door, but it can be gone just as fast, and then it's back to cleaning drains at the Esplanade.

I learned that I couldn't just be good. There are a lot of good actors out there. And there were certainly a lot of fresh-faced boys from middle America. I had to be as good as I could be. If I was worried about the money first, I wasn't going to give myself the best possible shot at getting the gig.

I attended acting classes at the Film Industry Workshop at the CBS Radford Studios in Studio City, and I would sing, in clubs or on friends' demo tapes, for no money. At auditions, I reminded myself I had to find the joy in this experience, because nobody was forcing me to do it. My parents offered to pay my college tab and I chose to do this instead, so shut up and read for Folgers. Bring the best coffee-loving face that Rob Paulsen has to offer. Leave it all on the casting room floor. I didn't want to be driving away and reading that line again and wishing I'd done it differently. You have one shot at these auditions, thirty seconds maybe. They're not going to let you turn around and do it again.

It was a cheap lesson. I can only imagine what real success might have done to me. If I had gotten a TV series at age twenty-five making $40,000 a week, maybe I would have done a bunch of blow, because that's what happened in the '80s. I might not have been able to handle it.

It was, unfortunately, a lesson I would again forget. Many years and many credits later, after an Emmy and a new house and a whole bunch of sports cars, the money bug bit me in the ass a second time. I had to once again navigate that line between what makes people want to buy you and not want to buy you.

That line is so sharp it'll cut you. And the wounds are much harder to heal when you're older.

But that was a future I could never imagine, focused as I was on the present. I'm happy to say that slowly I got my mind turned back around, and I rediscovered that joy. It was the passion, the obsession even, that drove me. I did it because I couldn't *not* do it.

I booked more commercials for Lee Jeans, Toyota, Ford, and Chevy. When I was out of my Jack in the Box commitment, I did McDonald's and KFC, then ventured into television shows and started getting more auditions for movie roles. I kept on hustling for work. I got a job on ABC's *New Love, American Style*, the daytime reboot of the popular 1970s comedy. *Love* only lasted a few months, crushed by competition from CBS's popular *The Price Is Right*, but I got to play a young husband in an episode with Sheila MacRae, who played the mother-in-law. This was my first big brush with fame.

The ex-wife of musical theater star Gordon MacRae, Sheila was a familiar face in our home as a regular on *The Red Skelton Hour* and *The Jackie Gleason Show*. She even appeared as herself on *I Love Lucy*. My parents were impressed that I shared the small screen with such a big celebrity, just as they were impressed when I met another Paulsen family favorite.

It was the mid-'80s and I was at the venerable Voicecaster studio in Burbank, auditioning for one thing or another, when I saw this lovely older woman at the pay phone telling AAA she had a flat tire.

When she hung up, I said, "Ma'am, if you have a spare, I can change the tire for you."

"Oh my gosh, young man, thank you. My car is parked out front."

I popped on the spare and rode with her to the garage to get a new tire. On the way back to the studio, she shook my hand and asked me my name again. I told her.

"Pleasure meeting you, Rob, my name is Gisele MacKenzie."

I had no idea. A Canadian singer, she had a big hit song in 1955 with "Hard to Get" and had appeared on TV shows starring Eddie Fisher, Dinah Shore, Pat Boone, and Ed Sullivan, but was most famous—at least at my house—for *Your Hit Parade* on TV.

When I called my dad later, he freaked out. I could hear him yelling to my mom, "Honey, Rob just changed Gisele MacKenzie's tire on Burbank Boulevard!"

I landed another one-episode gig, this time on *St. Elsewhere*, the hospital drama set in Boston, playing a Harvard frat boy named Ryan S. Hope who brought one of his buddies into the hospital after he got kneed in the groin while playing touch football. An examination determined the buddy had testicular cancer, and I spent the episode trying to deal with that fact.

The job reflected the unofficial way things work in Hollywood. I had actually read for another part on *St. Elsewhere* months earlier. The casting director was Eugene Blythe, who's beloved among actors because of his integrity. He called my agent to tell him that I was great at the read but not right for the part. I thought that was the end of it. But Gene remembered me, and when the frat kid role came along, he called me back in.

My biggest early acting experience gave me the chance to work with an honest-to-God auteur: Brian De Palma. I had seen *Scarface* and loved it. I thought of it as a cartoon Mafia cocaine movie. I had worked with his casting agent before, and while I didn't get the part on the earlier job, she called me back for what was described to me as a murder mystery thriller set in the porno movie industry that would be an homage to Alfred Hitchcock.

I read for a pretty good-size part. I walked into the room, and there was De Palma. He had on one of those khaki jackets that the new generation of directors—Kubrick, Coppola, Lucas, Spielberg—seemed to buy in bulk. I had heard that he liked to improvise. I liked to improvise. I read the lines as written, then went off script, and within moments, it seemed, the audition was over and I was back in my car on Santa Monica Boulevard.

Afterward, I made the long drive home. I was living near the beach in Oxnard, about sixty miles north, and when I got back, there was a message on my answering machine.

"He wants to use you," the casting agent said when I called back.

"What did I get?" I asked.

"You didn't get the part you read for. He really likes you, though. Three days' work next week in East Hollywood."

This was heaven. I had gotten a job in a Brian De Palma feature working with Craig Wasson and Melanie Griffith. The production team sent me what we call the sides—the pages of the script that are relevant to my character. They never want to release the whole script to secondary and tertiary characters.

The shoot took place in a large warehouse on Melrose in the eastern end of Hollywood. I parked out front near the production trucks and wardrobe trailers and checked in with the assistant director. I walked inside, and it was surreal. The set was closed to everybody but the actors, the AD, and De Palma.

The scene had us filming a movie within a movie, a porno flick called *Body Talk* set to the music of Frankie Goes to Hollywood. Dozens of extras were running around stark naked. I found out later that many of them were real adult film stars. Jack in the Box commercials were never like this.

I played a porno film cameraman who was filming a make-out session between Melanie Griffith, as porn starlet Holly Body, and Craig Wasson. Their make-out session left my character cold. I delivered my big lines: "Where's the cum shot? The cum shot! I thought we were doing *Body Talk* here, not *Last Tango*!"

Many years later, my son had friends over at the house one night watching movies on HBO. He was about fifteen or sixteen. I was in the other room taking a nap when I heard him call out to me.

"Hey, dad, were you in a movie called *Body Double*?"

Ah, the sins of the father.

CHAPTER FIVE

Welcome to Toontown

One day my agent called. "Rob, have you ever thought about doing cartoons?"

As a kid, I was a huge fan of *Looney Tunes*, and I knew all the names of the creators: the directors Bob Clampett and Chuck Jones, the animator Friz Freleng, the composers Carl Stalling and Milt Franklyn. I'd seen Mel Blanc on *The Tonight Show* just killing Johnny Carson. I knew a Bugs Bunny cartoon had won an Oscar. I loved how the music was a huge portion of the whole *Looney Tunes* world.

In high school, I started playing around with character voices and dialects in Mr. Lamb's basement studio. Because of his radio show and standing in the community, Mr. Lamb did a lot of commercials for Flint businesses, and his son Bob got to know a lot of these business owners.

We decided to try to find a way to do commercials with all this equipment. We wrote and produced them on spec in the hopes the shop owners would trade us stuff for commercials—I played golf and tennis and hockey and had a big need for stuff. We made a deal to do commercials for a company called Imperial Sports. In lieu of payment, they gave us tennis rackets, golf balls, and golf gloves.

I was a budding funny guy and used different voices in the commercials. We landed more partnerships, and soon I was hearing myself on Flint radio. Bob's younger brother Jeff became a successful DJ in Flint and a very talented voice guy in his own right. He created a late-night adult show called *Buffalo Dick's Radio Ranch*, and any time I went home to visit my parents, I would record bits for the show.

So I told my agent, sure, I'd be interested in cartoons, but I didn't have high hopes. In the early to mid-1980s, animation meant Saturday-morning cartoons on the three major networks. There was no Fox network, no cable channels, no direct to video. DVDs hadn't been invented yet.

The exceptions were the occasional after-school shows and the even more occasional prime-time series like *The Flintstones* and *Wait Till Your Father Gets Home*. Only two companies dominated animation, Disney and Hanna-Barbera. And only a small number of actors did the voices, and had done the voices, for decades. Others were famous or about to be famous. Don Adams from *Get Smart*, for example, also did Tennessee Tuxedo and Inspector Gadget.

I had done voice-over work for Jack in the Box and other commercials, but always in my own voice. My goal remained movies and music, though I wasn't averse to anything else. If I got a TV series, great. If I got a recording deal, great. If I became the new Dr Pepper guy, great. Animation could be part of that larger plan.

I had nothing against it. It just seemed like a pretty closed shop.

My agent said that Marvel Productions was coming up with new animated projects. Marvel in those days was not the movie behemoth it is now, with Iron Man and the Avengers. It was known for its comic books and Saturday morning cartoons. I didn't know much about Marvel. For all the cartoon work I would go on to do and all the Comic-Cons I'd attend, I was never much of a comic book guy. I liked some of them and read them. I knew who Stan Lee was. But I was never a comic collector. I mostly knew the Spider-Man cartoon, which started airing in the late 1960s, and its catchy theme song.

My agent told me the audition was for a new Marvel cartoon built around G.I. Joe. About three years earlier, Hasbro had relaunched their G.I. Joe toy line, with a new line called G.I. Joe: A Real American Hero, along with a new Marvel comic series. Hasbro partnered with Marvel to produce an animated show, essentially thirty-minute commercials for toys.

Like many boys, I had collected action figures for Major Matt

Mason, Trolls, Rat Fink. So of course, I had a G.I. Joe and all his different outfits and gear. I knew the theme song from the commercial. And I loved the military. My dad served in the Michigan National Guard for twenty years.

So I felt confident entering the world of G.I. Joe, as I walked into the audition at a studio on Hollywood Way, even if I knew nothing about the animation business. My introduction to this scene was the same as it was for all my Hollywood work: a nondescript room with chairs, music stands, microphones. I sat in the lobby with other actors and we were called in to read, back and forth, as they would mix and match us.

Probably the most common question I get asked is how I come up with the voices. This was something I learned on the job with *G.I. Joe*. It usually begins with drawings of the character, two-dimensional renderings on paper or, later in my career, three-dimensional computer-generated images. The drawings show different positions, attitudes, facial expressions. Then comes a written synopsis of the episode that explains the character's relationships to other characters in the story. This may also include any particular quirks the character has, catch-phrases, that sort of thing.

For *G.I. Joe*, they had me read for a newly created character called Snow Job, an alpine soldier who was all dressed in white, with white skis and a white rifle. I always thought it was a little odd that he also had a bright-red beard that would stand out in the snow. Any Russian sniper worth their salt could pick that guy off from three hundred yards.

They gave me four or five lines to read. The producers described Snow Job as coming from the Northeast, so I gave him a little Boston accent. Now, I've never been to Boston or known anybody who was from there. I ripped off the accent from memory, basing it on Walter Brennan on the old TV show *The Real McCoys*. Although Brennan's character, Grandpa Amos McCoy, was supposed to have come from deep in the Appalachian Mountains, the Massachusetts-born and -bred Brennan sounded like he'd just come off a lobster boat.

I asked myself, *How would Walter Brennan sound giving instructions on assembling a rifle?* I started riffing, flattening and stretching my As so that "car" became "caaaah" and "hockey" became "haaaawkey."

The producers seemed impressed, so they pushed me. They asked if

I was comfortable in a German dialect. In my early days, I said yes to everything, whether I could do it or not. Only later did I learn that you don't say yes to a voice unless you know you can kill it.

"Hey, do this one," a producer would say, and it was for a character with a Russian dialect. Or "Try this guy," he'd say. "He just crashed into the ocean and you need to make it sound like you're in the water."

Up to this point in my career, it was all about being the boy next door, your average-looking white kid. My agent would call and say the gig was for a guy between five foot nine and six feet tall who's at the beach, so wear a bathing suit to the audition. Other times they would be looking for a guy at a party, so I had to wear a tux. Same with voice-over work: I would be called upon to provide the nice, upbeat, generic smiley voice to sell the products, always in my own voice.

But reading Snow Job like a member of the Kennedy clan came as naturally to me as the first time I sang in a rock band in high school.

Would I have fooled a real-life Southie? Probably not, but I didn't have to. I just had to fool some cartoon producers in LA. And in that, I succeeded mightily. By the time I got home and called my agent, I had gotten the job. Taping began within days.

Then I called my parents, just as I did when I got the first Jack in the Box commercial, just as I did with every Hollywood job in those days.

"We love you," my dad would say. "Call us if you need anything, except for food, clothes, or money."

He was joking, but not entirely, and I never forgot what he'd said about me going into show business, and what he would have to tell his friends.

Each job proved him wrong.

When I walked into the studio for *G.I. Joe*, I didn't really know the actors with whom I was working. That is, I didn't know them by sight. But once they opened their mouths, it was overwhelming: Chris Collins, Arthur Burghardt, Michael Bell, Jack Angel, Frank Welker, all really wonderful actors who were profoundly gifted with their voices.

They could do anything, right there on the spot. Accents, dialects, sound effects. Cricket sounds, dogs, cats, monsters. Squirrels. I mean, what the hell does a squirrel sound like? They could pull off the craziest stuff.

In the beginning, the only actor on *G.I. Joe* I recognized was Frank

Welker, because I'd seen him on TV doing stand-up. He was a comic, a movie actor, and a master of impressions and sound effects. Frank used to regale us with stories from his movie days, telling us how Elvis Presley, during breaks while filming *Girls! Girls! Girls!*, would ask him over and over to do the sound of cats and dogs fighting.

During those first sessions for *G.I. Joe*, Frank messed around doing barks and chirps. Later, when I was working on a show called *Snorks*, which was essentially Smurfs underwater, the director asked Frank, "Give me a lobster sneezing underwater." Frank is one of the most accomplished voice actors in history. He's been both Scooby-Doo and Fred Jones. He's Abu the monkey in *Aladdin*, Garfield the cat, Oswald the Lucky Rabbit and Kermit the Frog as a baby. He's Nibbler on *Futurama*. He has a friggin' Emmy for lifetime achievement.

And damn if he couldn't sneeze like a submerged lobster.

Also on *G.I. Joe* was Peter Cullen, who played the master-of-camouflage assassin Zandar, rolling out his lines in a deep, mellifluous, overwhelming voice. Chris Collins, the Cobra Commander, did this hissing, evil-sounding thing on the spur of the moment. I became intoxicated by their voices and intimidated by the immediacy with which they could create characters, add nuance to a line, then change their voices completely, from snarling and raspy to the average guy next door. To play with these guys, to go from studio to studio, gig to gig, action figure to action figure, I realized I had to develop this kind of versatility. That would take time and dedication, and I was still on the fence about devoting myself to cartoons. I still held hope of making it as an on-camera actor.

While recording *G.I. Joe*, I continued to audition for TV and movies. As I mentioned, I had been sporting a mullet of various configurations, longer when I wasn't working, shortened when the job called for it. In those days, the most famous mullet in Hollywood belonged to Richard Dean Anderson, star of *MacGyver*, a show about a human superhero who possessed extraordinary powers of tinkering, solving huge problems with small objects, like hot-wiring a fighter jet with a rusted paper clip.

It was a really huge show, one of ABC's top-rated prime-time series for years, and in 1985 I scored a guest spot in an episode about a little girl who accesses a NORAD missile base via her Commodore computer. I was an FBI agent who had to assist MacGyver in figuring out who this girl was and how to stop her.

When I came on set and saw the other guest actor I'd be working with, I gasped, "That's the Professor!"

Two decades later, he had put on some pounds and of course wasn't wearing those island khakis, but I recognized him instantly. Russell Johnson from *Gilligan's Island* had been cast as my boss, the more seasoned FBI agent.

I was tongue-tied. *Gilligan's Island* was an iconic TV show, airing for only three seasons but living on forever in reruns I used to watch back in Michigan. I didn't know what he'd be like in real life. Like many, I had also heard the cautionary tales about how some of the cast wound up bitter, having made a mint for the producers but getting no residuals for all those reruns.

I introduced myself, and Russell couldn't have been nicer. We were chatting on set, and I finally got up the nerve to ask, "What's it like to be part of television history?"

"It's good and bad," Russell said. He was referring to the fact that he never made much money from the show, without the rerun residuals.

"On the other hand, young man," said Russell, "my wife and I just got back from a trip to the British Isles and spent weeks visiting different abbeys, and every single one of the brothers knew who I was. That's a gift I will always have. Nobody will ever be able to take it away from me."

What's more, he said, he was still able to work as an actor, thanks to his *Gilligan* fame. "And I'm grateful for that."

I promised myself that if I ever made even half the impact on popular culture that these actors did, I'd try to be like the Professor.

One of my biggest commercial gigs earlier in my career was for Crush International, the company that made a drink called Sundrop, a Mountain Dew–like soda sold primarily in the Southeast. My buddy Jeff Harlan and I had been hired for a series of TV, radio, and print ads about two young brothers on the road to Nashville.

We were on location in North Carolina, where Sundrop was widely consumed, to shoot commercials shot at Catawba County Fair in Hickory, North Carolina. After meeting the local crew, Jeff and I—the "LA talent"—went to the hotel.

There in the lobby was a stunningly beautiful brunette with white skin like alabaster. It didn't take long before we started talking to her. She was a local girl named Parrish, working as a production coordinator on the shoot, and we both had an immediate crush on her.

Fortunately, she decided I was the lesser of two evils and took pity on me. She moved out to Los Angeles, we started dating, and in 1984 we got married. We had rented a little house on the beach in Oxnard, which is where we were sitting when I saw the first episode of *G.I. Joe: A Real American Hero.*

Even though I had only a few lines, it was a whole different experience than seeing myself in my little Jack in the Box hat and name tag. In some ways it exceeded working on a De Palma set. With this little role, in which nobody saw my face, I had become more than a working actor. I was now a part of the legacy of a show. I was part of *G.I. Joe.* It was not going to go away like Frings.

When I was a kid, I would watch cartoons that were made in the 1940s and '50s. They're forever. Now there was going to be some other little kid watching this show I was in, and I was part of it, part of the permanence and the relevance. Of all of the acting jobs I had scored since coming out to Hollywood, this represented the strongest reinforcement that leaving Michigan, leaving the band, leaving my friends and family, was the right thing to do. And I had my own action figure: Snow Job in a bubble-wrap package.

Legacy meant something more to me for other reasons. My wife was now pregnant.

Around this time I shot a TV pilot in Texas, just outside Dallas, for a series envisioned as a sort of *Three's Company* meets *Bosom Buddies.* Both were hit shows, and in Hollywood imitation is the highest form of laziness.

Nothing ever happened with the show—the network didn't pick up the pilot, which is not uncommon. A lot of actors scratch out careers shooting pilots nobody ever sees. But the casting director remembered me and knew I could pull off that crazy, over-the-top stuff, so she called me in to read for a movie.

These were the heady years after *Porky's*, when every TV network was cranking out *Animal House* knockoffs and every movie producer was looking for R-rated comedies. The film was called *Stewardess School*, and the title pretty much says it all: *Police Academy* in the air.

The role was for a character named Larry Falkwell, a stereotypical, flamboyantly gay flight attendant. Nothing about the character as written was terribly deep. He was gay, funny, and resourceful. He could disarm a bomb with a bobby pin. The casting director, having seen my work on the pilot, knew that I would swing for the fences, which is what I did at the audition. I pulled out everything I had, improvising on set, holding nothing back. And I got the part.

One of the film's stars was Donny Most from *Happy Days*, which had just ended its phenomenal run on ABC about a year earlier. Another actor was Brett Cullen, a great guy and wonderful actor who'd already done the miniseries *The Thorn Birds* and went on to a prolific career that included *Lost*, *Ghost Rider*, *Person of Interest*, and *Narcos*. One of the actresses was Mary Cadorette, who had just come off the *Three's Company* spin-off *Three's a Crowd*. And the featured actor was George Jefferson himself, Sherman Hemsley.

I knew going into this that the film was no *Citizen Kane*. The film was a bomb. Released in 1986, it brought in $136,158, landing it at number 10,520 on the all-time domestic gross list. It may be one of the worst-performing movies of all time. It was, in short, not a good movie in my opinion.

Fans occasionally ask me today why on earth I took that job. I did it for the same reasons I take roles today: it's work. I'm in a better position today to behave with a little more discretion, which I even exercise on occasion, but I still like to work, and this movie, for all its faults, was a big step up for me. *Stewardess School* offered me a second-banana role. I'd be in all the cast photos, get third or fourth billing on the credits, and have my own (temporary) parking space at the studio, the opportunity to work with real pros, and a nice paycheck, which I badly needed. Our son, Ashton, had been born a few months earlier, and I needed money for diapers.

My folks and my wife's mother would come out for two or three weeks at a time to watch Ash. During one such trip, I brought my mother to the *Stewardess School* set. She was a big fan of *The Jeffersons*, and Sherman Hemsley could not have been sweeter. He took the time to make a fuss over my mother. As I was getting coffee, I could hear Sherman say, "Where's Lee at? Where's my girlfriend?" My mother beamed at the attention.

For a young actor on his first feature film, this was all a dream. It was a twelve-week shoot at the Warner Bros. lot, which would play such a huge part in my life later on with *Animaniacs*. I was playing with people who were above my pay grade, in money and talent and celebrity. They could have hired Scott Baio, but they hired me. I had cracked the ceiling just a little bit.

Those were different times, times when cheap, prejudiced stereotypes ran rampant in entertainment. I wouldn't even audition for the Larry character today. At the same time, I don't apologize for it. The goal was to make the role funny, not offensive. Bottom line: I was hired, I did it, and I own it.

As much as I loved movie acting, it took a toll on my family life. At the time of the shoot, we lived right on the beach, renting a two-bedroom bungalow in Oxnard, about sixty miles northwest of Los Angeles. Living so far from LA meant we could afford to have the sand in our backyard. But it made for a drive of up to two hours each way in traffic to the Warner Bros. lot in Burbank.

I had so much fun at work that I felt guilty each night when I came home. My wife would be understandably exhausted from the baby, and I worried that she'd resent the fact I spent my days goofing around on a movie set. As much as I was having a ball, I felt like I had to put a lid on how exciting my day was. I didn't want to rub it in. This was the first time I had to deal with leaving my wife and my new son at home for so long. Depending on how my career went, I realized, it wouldn't be the last. If I were to continue with feature films, which had more demanding work schedules and often required extended travel to film on location, this would become the new normal.

But luckily, while trying to make a go of it as a movie star, I continued to snap up work as a voice actor for cartoons—work that was turning into a love affair. After *G.I. Joe*, cartoon people were starting to take notice of this guy Rob Paulsen: Hey, he's pretty clever. He can change his voice. Oh, it turns out he can sing, too, and sing in character. And we don't care if he's six foot two or two foot six, black, white, green, or orange, mullet or no mullet. He's not afraid to play.

I was watching these guys during the *G.I. Joe* sessions in awe. And they were just in T-shirts and baseball hats. I was in Hollywood heaven. I had found my home. "Please, please, please," I said to my agent, "send me as much animation as you can. I want to do cartoons."

The *G.I. Joe* director, Wally Burr, helped me land a job for another Marvel show. I had no idea what that show was about, except that it was based on action figures that I had never heard of or seen. I did a few small roles, characters called Slingshot and Air Raid, both cocky, Top Gun–type fighter pilots.

Who knew that a couple decades later this show would be part of a multibillion-dollar franchise known as *Transformers*. To this day, people still have me sign action figures. Back then, I just wanted to work with this great group of actors who would become my friends: Frank Welker again, this time voicing Megatron, and Peter Cullen, who was the voice of Optimus Prime.

The studio that every voice actor coveted was Hanna-Barbera. At the time it was still independently owned. It traced its cartoon roots to before World War II, when William Hanna and Joseph Barbera collaborated at MGM on *Tom and Jerry*. For nearly twenty years, they made MGM cartoon shorts before forming their own studio in 1957, located in the old Charlie Chaplin studios on La Brea.

Hanna-Barbera had one hit after another: *The Huckleberry Hound Show*, *The Yogi Bear Show*, *Quick Draw McGraw*, *The Flintstones*, and the original *Scooby Doo, Where Are You!* By the 1970s they were churning out Saturday-morning cartoons the way Detroit rolled out Fords: *Josie and the Pussycats*; *Inch High, Private Eye*; *Valley of the Dinosaurs*; shows based on the Harlem Globetrotters; and many incarnations of their biggest property, *Scooby-Doo*. They fed shows to all three networks and to countries around the world, and in 1981 they had another blockbuster show in *The Smurfs*, with its lucrative merchandising.

If Hanna-Barbera was the voice acting holy grail, then the person everybody wanted to work for was director Gordon Hunt. His credits included everything from *The Jetsons* to *Scooby-Doo*. Gordon had a background in theater with a reputation as a world-class acting coach. After working as a freelance director in New York, he served as casting director at the Mark Taper Forum in LA for a decade before he went to Hanna-Barbera.

To be on a Gordon Hunt show at Hanna-Barbera as an actor was like a stand-up comic getting on *The Tonight Show*. As my animation career began to take off, I did a general audition at Hanna-Barbera in the hopes of working for him someday. They gave me four or five pieces of copy to see what I could do. Some bits were funny, some serious, some in dialects. I did some sound effects that I had been working on since watching my impressive *G.I. Joe* costars. I sang in character.

The veteran actors motivated me. I had listened to Peter Cullen and had practiced lowering my high tenor to a tough-guy growl. I could effect a lot of this through microphone technique. When I brought my mouth closer to the mic, I could create that deeper, more sinister tone. But if I got too close, my *p*'s would pop and send the recording levels haywire. The trick was to "boom" without popping and overmodulating. I bought a cheap Radio Shack cassette player and practiced my mic axis at home. Before long, I could boom with the best of them.

I was soon called in to read for one of Hanna-Barbera's biggest new shows, a reboot of *Jonny Quest*. Inspired by radio dramas and several adventure comic books, the original show became one of those rare animated series to air in prime time when it debuted on ABC in 1964. Drawn with a realistic look unusual for television animation, the show followed the towheaded Jonny Quest and his scientist father through jungle adventures. The original show lasted all of one season but lived on for decades in reruns, which was how I had seen it as a kid.

In 1986, I read for Hadji, the turbaned East Indian boy whose catch phrase is "Sim Sim Salabim." Hadji would make cool stuff happen, hopefully in the nick of time, so that Jonny, Race, Dr. Quest, and Bandit the dog would not fall into the nefarious hands of some crazy mad scientist.

They wanted me to pretty much do what had been done in the original by a kid actor named Danny Bravo, who had small roles in movies and TV shows in the 1960s. I listened to audio recording examples and it didn't take me long to nail it, because I was a big fan of that show and knew the voice well. Soon I, too, was dashing off

"Sim Sim Salabim" and "Careful, there's a pterodactyl!" in a vaguely Indian accent.

Don Messick reprised his Dr. Quest role, which was mind-blowing. When I first walked into the room and he opened his mouth, it transported me back to Detroit at ten years old. He did the voice of Boo Boo and the Ranger on *Yogi Bear*. He played Papa Smurf on *The Smurfs*, and originated the voice of Scooby-Doo, which Frank Welker would later take over. Don was a remarkable talent, one of those old-school guys with a long career we all envied.

They hired a new Jonny Quest, a terrific actor named Scott Menville, who'd go on to enjoy a great career that had him doing everything from Fred Flintstone and Shaggy in reboots of *The Flintstones* and *Scooby-Doo* to a variety of voices in *Avatar: The Last Airbender* and the *Spider-Man* cartoon.

I got the freakin' job on *Jonny Quest*. And I was going to be directed by none other than Gordon Hunt. It was a turning point in my career, starring in the reprisal of a very significant show in the lives of millions of little kids who were born in the '50s and '60s. It would be a big deal to them, just like it was to me. And I was thrilled to have a steady job—thirteen half-hour episodes at about eight hundred bucks a pop. I had a new baby and rent and car payments. I was doing the math in my head and said, *Holy smoke, I'm guaranteed ten grand!* I was being treated like a real Hollywood player.

I drove up to the gate of the studios on Cahuenga Boulevard, and the guard greeted me by name.

"How you doing there, Robbie?"

"Great, uh—"

"Call me Bobby. Everybody calls me Bobby. Go ahead, Robbie. Off you go."

I didn't have to worry about my ID, because he knew who I was. As I walked into the building, everything I saw was Flintstones and Smurfs, Huckleberry Hound and Quick Draw McGraw. It was literally walls covered with memories of my childhood. I would wander around in a stupor the first few times I went.

Hadji became my calling card. I had something that my agent could cite for auditions. Casting agents would say, "I'm sorry, we don't know who this kid is," and my agent could tell them, "Yeah, well, he's now the voice of Hadji on *Jonny Quest.*" *Bring him in* was the response. If he's good enough for Gordon Hunt, he's good enough for us.

From an acting standpoint, it gave me the opportunity to work not only with Gordon but with this parade of incredible guest stars who came from that generation of actors, all now in their '60s and '70s, who started out as radio stars and had transitioned into voice work, just like Mel Blanc.

Jonny Quest and other Hanna-Barbera shows also introduced me to the cream of the character actor crop: Hamilton Camp, Bob Ridgely, Jack Riley, Bill Daily, Marcia Wallace, Arte Johnson, Ruth Buzzi, Henry Gibson—people I grew up watching on network television, on prime-time sitcoms. They were part of *Rowan & Martin's Laugh-In* and *The Bob Newhart Show.* They were part of *Petticoat Junction* or *Green Acres.* And I was at the next microphone.

I came to admire and learn from their courage, which they drew from Gordon Hunt. Gordon loved actors. He encouraged everybody. All these celebrities, these seminal figures in my childhood, were encouraged to access their creativity. He didn't want them to just stick to the script. These veteran actors would dive in. No matter how famous they were, they were not afraid to look bad, not afraid to try silly stuff. They showed no self-consciousness. Much of this was because nobody could see them. There would be old women, young men, heavy people, thin people, people who were hired for on-air work for the way they looked. But in here, they could be anybody.

Sometimes I would see people my parents' age behaving in this really outrageous way—Carol Channing, John Astin, and Rip Taylor, all making blue jokes and bouncing off the walls and being very sweet and incredibly generous to a kid like me. They offered tips and guidance and encouragement, but most of all, inspiration.

They had mastered the art of unlearning adult behaviors. Some of them were raunchy, in the down-and-dirtiest, Lenny Bruce and Rusty Warren sense. We'd be doing a children's show and every other word off-mic is "fuck this" or "fuck that."

Carol Channing, who worked with me on another show, would come in and jokingly say something like, "I bet you never seen an ass like mine."

Offended? Hell no. She's Carol Channing. She's a theater dame. When you see that at twenty-seven years old, you think, "Well, then, man, if Ms. Channing responds to that, maybe I can be that way, too."

So I would join in. It was a fraternity of whack jobs, and I was a new pledge. They'd give me a hug and say, "Gosh, you're doing a great job, Ron," and I wouldn't have the guts to correct them.

The new *Jonny Quest* lasted no longer than the original. After one year and thirteen episodes, we were done by 1987. But Gordon noticed my fearlessness and would bring me in for more and more shows. Soon I became a guest on a number of series. Then I would get leads alongside bona fide stars.

When Hanna-Barbera produced an animated version of *The Addams Family*, John Astin reprised the TV role he made famous as Gomez. Uncle Fester was played by Rip Taylor, whom I'd seen every day on *Hollywood Squares*. Grandmama was Carol Channing, and Lurch was my buddy Jim Cummings.

The cartoon added two characters. They were going to be like the Kravitzes on *Bewitched*—nosy neighbors who'd watch the strange goings on from across the street. They were Mr. and Mrs. Normanmeyer. I was cast as Mr. Normanmeyer and my wife was played by Edie McClurg, a wonderful comic actress trained in the Groundlings comedy troupe. The show was another big boost to my career and had a profound personal impact: John Astin became a good friend to me, and his son Sean would become one of my closest pals.

———

For a guy who never went to church much, religion would play a big role in my career. And I don't just mean the Covenant Players. Hanna-Barbera's cofounder Joe Barbera was a devout Catholic who aspired to do a series called *The Greatest Adventure: Stories from the Bible*. It would feature three young time travelers sent through a portal into different biblical tales, teaching them lessons they may not have appreciated from the page. As powerful as Hanna-Barbera was in Hollywood, no network would touch a show with such overtly Christian material.

So Mr. Barbera decided to take the then-novel step of releasing it directly to video.

One of the time travelers was Moki, a boy with an Indian accent, and Mr. Barbera asked, "Hey, who's that kid we got doing Hadji?"

"That's Rob Paulsen," he was told.

"Get him in here. He sounds like he could do this."

The next thing I knew, I was working with disc jockey–turned–actor Terry McGovern and singer-actress Darleen Carr, dashing off to cartoon Babylon, Mount Ararat, and Nazareth. We were the regulars and each week had A-list guest stars. Lorne Greene from *Bonanza* was Noah and James Earl Jones played a pharaoh.

As usual, Gordon directed. One day, he brought in his daughter, this wonderful young upstart actress. I thought, "She's really good."

The rest of Hollywood would also think so. His daughter is Helen Hunt.

After that, I voiced minor characters on *The Smurfs* and its aquatic version, *Snorks*, in which I voiced Corky the Snork, who sounds like an extra in *Waiting for Guffman*. I worked with Nancy Cartwright, who's Bart on *The Simpsons*.

When I wasn't at the Hanna-Barbera studios, I was at NBC doing a Saturday-morning cartoon show called *Fraggle Rock*. It featured the Muppets in animated form. It was like everything else Jim Henson did: excellent. I played Boober, who was a—now I think about it, I don't know what Boober was. Or what a Fraggle was. Boober had a Kermit the Frog/Ray Romano voice. I also played a dog called Sprocket that went "roo-roo." The third character was Marjory the Trash Heap, the first and only talking heap of trash I've ever done. It was also my first female voice. I gave Marjory a nondescript Eastern European accent.

It never occurred to me to question whether the Fraggles could talk. Of course they could. That's why I loved this form of acting—the unfettered creativity, the opportunity to try anything. In a few short years, I had gone from admiring the versatility of my costars to being able, in one show, to pull off a rock, a dog, and a pile of trash.

I was starting to make some nice bucks. Between day rates and residuals, I was approaching $100,000 a year. That was a lot of bread for a guy who'd just turned thirty, more money in a year than my father ever made selling auto supplies. I had come out to Los Angeles to pursue fame and fortune. The fortune part seemed like it was working out.

But the trade-off was that I'd be walking down the street and nobody would recognize me. I had friends in stand-up comedy getting on *The Tonight Show*, other friends landing sitcoms. My buddy Phil Hartman had just booked *Saturday Night Live*. I was earning good money, but on kid shows.

Sometimes, feeling envious, I would question whether cartoons would be enough for me. But all of that was about to change.

One day, the *Fraggle Rock* director, Stu Rosen, came into the studio and told us about a new cartoon in the works based on a comic book. The drawings were in black-and-white, and it had a big underground following.

He told us the name. For all the animated shows I'd done, as I said, I'm really not a comic book guy. I had never heard of this one.

"What's it about?" I asked Stu.

"Turtles," he said.

CHAPTER SIX

Cowabunga!

It was much darker on the page. Kevin Eastman and Peter Laird imagined Raphael as an assassin. The other guys were badasses, too. "We're going to fight the forces of darkness," they said. It was intense and weird, a twisted parody of four popular comics of the day: *The New Mutants*, *Daredevil*, *Cerebus*, and *Ronin*.

At the time of the audition, I knew none of this. I read with another *Fraggle Rock* actor, Townsend Coleman, and all we knew was that the characters were turtles named after Renaissance artists and each had a distinct personality. And they lived in a sewer and fought like ninjas.

In the cartoon business, this all made perfect sense. From what the producers told me, Raphael was kind of a caustic smart-ass. I'm pretty good at that, so I read for him in my own voice. Mikey was the happy-go-lucky party dude, the "cowabunga" guy, and Townie tried out for him.

The audition came as my career had hit a crossroads. I was having a blast doing animation but was still trying to squeeze in on-camera work, *Body Double* and *Stewardess School* having left me with hopes of a film career.

While in the midst of my Hanna-Barbera work, my agent called: "Listen, they want to see you for *Hill Street Blues*. You're a junkie father. Dress casual."

"Okay," I said. "When is that?"

"It's tomorrow, two fifteen, over at NBC."

"I can't."

"You can't?" My agent was incredulous. *Hill Street Blues* was one of the hottest shows on TV, a prime-time hit.

"The problem is," I said, "I'm working on *Jonny Quest* from ten to one, and then from two to six, I'm working on *The Addams Family*."

"Cartoons?" my agent said. "This is NBC."

I didn't want to aggravate my agent or alienate NBC. But I also didn't want to ask the folks at Hanna-Barbera, "Would you mind if I came in two hours late?" Of course they'd mind. They weren't going to change the schedule to accommodate my fledgling TV career. Make too many of those kinds of demands, and I'd start losing cartoon gigs.

One of my mentors at Hanna-Barbera was an actor named Alan Oppenheimer. We worked together on the Bible show, and he was such a versatile talent that in different episodes he played Noah, one of the wise men, and King Belshazzar. Alan is in his late eighties now and one of my closest friends. I told him my issues with my agent and my struggle with turning down on-camera work.

"You know what, young man, you're going to have to make a decision, because you're pretty good at this. Gordon likes you.

"You're not afraid to be bad," he continued. "You're not afraid to try stuff. You can take a good ribbing when you do something stupid and silly. You can take it. You might really want to think about devoting your energy to this."

At the *Turtles* audition, the producers narrowed the cast down to four actors and had us all read for other parts. Barry Gordon first gave Michelangelo a shot, but Donatello was the turtle for him. Barry is a wonderful actor, who has that nerdy, nebbishy voice that worked better for Donatello, who was written as a sort of geeky gadget guy. Cam Clarke did Leonardo in a clear, heroic voice, lending the gravitas he had from years in show business as a former child performer who grew up before our eyes on *The King Family Show*; his mother was one of the King Sisters.

It came down to a toss-up between Townie and me for Michelangelo and Raphael. Michelangelo is the party dude, and try as I did, I couldn't match Townie, who gave him that crazy surfer affectation. The truth is Raphael, cool but crude, always was the best fit for me.

We're both smart-asses, so I decided not to do an accent, dialect, or any other kind of affectation. I didn't change my voice, and they didn't want me to change my voice. They wanted me to fire up my sarcastic side, and I got the job.

The producers explained that the show was going to be a five-episode arc, paid for by Playmates Toys, which had licensed the characters to make action figures. It was going to be syndicated by Group W television. If the show did well, there could be more episodes. Our expectations were modest.

Our first recording sessions were an absolute blast. I had known Townie from *Fraggle Rock* and other shows. We both had that all-American look and often ran into each other at auditions for on-camera gigs. I had worked with the director Stu Rosen for years at Hanna-Barbera. With Barry and Cam, it was like we were brothers. We opened our scripts and all looked at each other and said, this *Turtles* thing is crazy enough that it just might work.

Since this was a brand-new show, the producers gave us the Turtle backstory and ethos. They told us how the four turtles got hit with this ooze and took on the characteristics of the last animal they were in touch with: in this case, humans. The leader, Splinter, was a ninja who also came in contact with the ooze and took on the characteristics of a rat. The leader had a deep love of Renaissance art and took on these turtles as his children, naming them after famous artists. It was a complicated, interesting backstory, nothing that I'd ever experienced before in animation.

But what became apparent from the start was the theme of family. I had worked on ensemble casts before—*G.I. Joe, Transformers*—but *Turtles* possessed such a deep and poignant feeling of brotherhood. We were like Frankenstein monsters and babes in the woods, living below the surface, looking out for each other.

When I think about other shows I'd worked on to that point, nothing had such a direct emphasis on family. We fought like brothers, but we were taking care of each other. We were literally our brothers' keepers. Pretty heavy stuff in the context of a cartoon show.

What was also interesting was that, while we had these ninja skills and could fight like crazy, nobody ever died. If anything got busted, it was a machine or robots. There was more humor than in the comic books, with these wiseacre, pizza-eating "heroes in a half shell." It was sweet and smart and deep and clever, kid- and family-friendly.

The show came out for the 1987 Christmas TV break. It did okay. It didn't do great guns, just well enough for producers to green-light eight more episodes. That would bring the total to the magic thirteen so they could "strip them," meaning they could run the episodes four times over a fifty-two-week cycle.

The extra episodes meant more time in the studio and more awkward phone calls with my agent. I turned down that NBC audition; there were a hundred other guys like me that *Hill Street Blues* could cast. The show would survive without me. But how many other actors could help bring to life a turtle with ninja skills? I kept returning in my mind to that conversation with Allen. I did have to make a decision. Cartoons grabbed me like nothing else had before.

The question was whether my ego could handle the fact that nobody was going to know what I looked like.

As the animation work piled up, I struggled to slip away for TV and movie auditions. If I couldn't squeeze in a quick reading, there was no way I could also juggle a guest spot on a TV show, much less a movie role. I was still making that punishing commute from LA to Oxnard. As my son started toddling around that cramped beach house, with my wife at home all day without any help from me, simmering marital tensions began to boil into arguments.

Finally, we left the beach. In the winter of 1986, we moved into a West Hollywood apartment building that looked like something out of *Miami Vice*. It was painted salmon pink with teal-green trim. I felt like I was living in Don Johnson's clothes. The hope was that putting me closer to the studios would relieve some of that pressure at home. But even shaving two hours off my commute didn't give me enough time for everything I was trying to do: animation recording and auditions. And always that dream of getting a movie role—a job that would keep me away from my family even more. We next moved into another place, a duplex in Hollywood. That gave us more space but didn't solve my career question—or give my wife hope that I wouldn't be dashing off to a film location at the spur of the moment.

Finally she said, "Don't take this the wrong way—I think you're good-looking, but maybe voice acting is best for you."

When she met me, I was an on-camera actor; she knew how important that was for me. But by now she'd also met my colleagues. I'd stood there as Gordon Hunt told her how I was a natural in the recording studio. "He's sliding into this and that. He's killing it," he'd gushed.

So maybe, she said, I could have a different kind of fame, the kind that satisfied me creatively, that made a good living but also got me home at a decent hour. I wouldn't get approached by fans in a restaurant, but neither, she noted, would our son. We could have a regular life, and I could still work in Hollywood.

I chuckled. "Maybe I do have a face for cartoons."

Parrish was right. Of course.

That year, 1988, *Ninja Turtles* exploded. The world couldn't get enough of these guys, and everybody was now shouting, "Turtle power!"

Everything about the Turtles was atypical. Normally a show starts out on a network then goes into syndication. But as *Turtles* got bigger and bigger in syndication, it was picked up by a network, CBS. In those days, I was too close to it to realize what was happening. We were cloistered in the studio, doing voices, tossing ideas back and forth, just trying to bring life to the Turtles.

I always knew that when my parents would call me about something I was doing, it was a big deal.

"What are they, lizards?" my dad asked.

"It's *Ninja Turtles*," I said.

"All I know," he said, "is that the guys I work with, my God, their kids and their grandkids, they're losing their minds over this thing."

I said, "That's my voice."

"Now, which one are you?" he asked. "What's special about you?"

"Dad, you wouldn't get it."

A short time later, the phone rang again.

"Hi, honey, it's Mom. I'm sorry, I hate to do this, but one of the principals found out that I was your mom, and, well, would you mind doing a favor?"

My mom was working at the school district at the time and said, "The principal wanted to know if you could call their grandkids in that Turtle voice."

"Mind?" I said. "I'd love to!"

My parents had seen me on TV before, in the commercials, on *MacGyver* and *New Love, American Style,* and my mom had even been on the *Stewardess School* set, but this was the first project where they would tell people, "My kid is famous—sort of."

I never forgot that my parents had both expressed concerns about my dropping out of college and moving to Los Angeles. While my mom was still supportive, despite her reservations, my father had asked me over and over, "What the hell are you doing?"

I was ecstatic that, with the Turtles, I finally did something my parents were proud of. It was the first of several projects in which I could remind them, subtly—and sometimes not so subtly—that I wasn't as stupid as I seemed.

When my parents came out to LA to visit in 1989, right after I had bought a new home with my animation money, my father offered what I took to be his attempt at an apology.

"Well, you sure showed me," he said, then asked me how much I paid for the house. I told him $572,000.

"Jesus Christ," he said. "The home you were raised in, I paid $40,000."

As I was getting ready to leave the house for an animation gig, I donned my usual uniform: T-shirt, jeans, baseball hat.

My father asked, "You're going to work like that? In a baseball hat?" He was a steel salesman. He always wore a buttoned shirt and tie.

"I'll probably turn it around when I record," I said, "because I don't want it to interfere with the microphone."

I think there was this moment when they had to reconcile that their oldest kid was making a good living doing essentially what got him into trouble at the dinner table.

For years afterwards, as I moved from *Turtles* to *Animaniacs,* my dad used to play the semicelebrity card often. During one visit to Michigan, I was home only half an hour before my dad mentioned some buddy on the street whose seventeen-year-old daughter was interested in show business.

"I told him you'd take her out to lunch," my dad said.

"Uh, do you think that's appropriate?" I said.

"Oh, yeah, her mom and dad are fine with it. Take her out to lunch. Make her feel special. It's okay, her dad's chief of police."

I opted to just chat with her at our house.

Likewise, when we went to a Mexican restaurant in Gaylord, Michigan, called La Señorita, my dad went up to the hostess and said, "You ever watch the *Ninja Turtles*?"

She probably thought my dad had had a few pops before he got there. I rescued him and said, "I make my living doing cartoon voices."

"Are you kidding?" she said.

"Why would I make that up?" I said. "If I was going to lie to you about being famous, I'd say that I was Brad Pitt's half brother."

Then my dad said, "You ever watch *Pinky and the Brain*? He does all those, too."

It's relative celebrity. In northern Michigan, a retired football player for the Lions is a celebrity. But it was a big deal for my parents.

My mother usually never pulled the semicelebrity card unless it was clandestine, asking me to call a neighbor's friend's nephew and record a voice mail in a cartoon voice. But if we had an autograph signing in the Midwest, my parents would come and visit my coworkers and me. Then it would be in full swing. The crowd was there, and my parents could revel in it and say, "That's my kid."

During one signing, my mom sat quietly to the side and watched, her hands folded in her lap, smiling the whole time. I went over and gave my mom a big hug and told the fans who she was. Then out of the blue, somebody asked her for an autograph.

She blushed and said, "Oh my gosh, I'm nobody."

I said, "No, you aren't. You're Pinky's mom."

I was also a big hit at my son's school. I'm not going to lie: I think I looked forward to career day at his elementary school more than the Emmy awards. Each year, the teacher would introduce the other parents and what they did for a living—the doctor, the lawyer, the investment banker.

Then the teacher would say, "And here's Ash's dad. He's Raphael!" And the kids would go insane.

And every year, one of Ash's classmates would call him at home. I'd overhear Ash say, "Yes, Jason, he really is. No, really." Then he'd hand me the phone: "Dad, Jason wants to talk to Raphael."

I would go, "Cowabunga, dude!" and then hand the phone back to Ash.

"See, Jason, I told you."

The best experience with my parents came in 2000, just before my parents' fiftieth wedding anniversary. My father was involved in the alumni association of the Howe Military School. A lot of the teachers there were of the age that they had grown up watching cartoons I'd done. I was invited to give a talk at the school. I answered questions, sang "Yakko's World," and signed autographs. They made me an honorary military captain and gave me a fancy plaque.

And I could tell, my father finally understood why it meant so much to me. I'm sure he had made a big fuss over me before I got there. He now could share in the experience. Now, I know a person qualifies as a celebrity in northern Michigan for winning best pig at the county fair.

But on this day, for his purposes, I was Laurence Olivier.

Although we were only the actors on *Ninja Turtles*, we felt we had a big role in making the characters who they were and, therefore, a big part of the show's success. We ended up doing nine years and almost two hundred episodes. It went from literally a clean sheet of paper to one of the biggest, if not the biggest, animation/toy franchises of all time, up there with Barbie, Transformers, and the Disney characters.

In making any animated show, we record the lines first, and then the artists get to work. The beauty of doing it this way is that you're not limited by being locked into the pictures. This is the time to try stuff. It doesn't work that way in on-camera jobs, where you'd be burning all kinds of daylight and wasting the time of a lot of crew members by messing around.

Animation is the ultimate playground. It's the ultimate sandbox for an actor.

We were encouraged to be what we wanted to be on *Turtles*. We improvised all the time. We would encourage each other. "Try this. It might be kind of funny," we'd say. Sometimes it made it into the show, many times it didn't. It was egoless.

That's not to say that egos can't be bruised.

We never got officially informed that they would be making a feature film based on the show. The news was just kind of around town. I probably saw it in *Variety* or the *Hollywood Reporter*. The production company for the movie had nothing to do with the animation company I worked with. The characters were licensed by Mirage Studios, which was created by Eastman and Laird.

And the producers hired different actors as the Turtles. I never even had a chance to audition. My guy, Raphael, was played by Josh Pais. You've seen Josh over the years on scores of TV shows, from *Law & Order: Special Victims Unit* to *Ray Donovan*. At the time, he was an unknown actor with a couple of TV credits and no cartoon voice experience.

The film *Teenage Mutant Ninja Turtles* came out in 1990, while we were at the peak of our run with the cartoon. The cartoon clearly inspired the look and vibe of the movie, at least partially, the Turtles cracking wise as they emerged from the New York sewers to take on the Foot Clan and save the skin of reporter April O'Neil.

"What the hell," one of my *Turtle* cast mates said. "I thought they would use us."

We weren't angry so much as surprised, and I think a little hurt. Maybe *hurt* is too strong a word. We were disappointed. People don't always believe me when I say this, but it never went beyond that. I didn't see anybody on the cast get their noses out of joint.

This was one of those moments when a voice actor has to come to grips with his or her place in Hollywood. We realized that as hard as we worked on the voices, the show wasn't about how we, specifically, did the Turtles. Other characters—Mickey Mouse, say—have an iconic, specific, recognizable voice. Disney treats it as such. That's why they have one guy, maybe two, to do Mickey all the time. They always stay on point.

The same thing with *The Simpsons*. When many of the *Simpsons* actors had to withhold their services in 1998 because they wanted to get a little more dough, the producers threatened to recast, and it was a disaster. Fox ultimately stayed with the regular actors (and gave them raises) because, I'm convinced, it was established and the audience would know the difference.

We didn't have that with the *Turtles*. The fact is, when the movie came out, I don't recall any eleven-year-old saying, "I'm not watching this because Rob Paulsen isn't in it."

My own son was all about the *Turtles* movie. He played the video games. We used to go to arcades and get a pile of quarters and spend the afternoon playing *Ninja Turtles*. He was dying to see the movie when it came out. And he didn't give a shit that I wasn't in it.

Financed independently and shot in North Carolina, doubling as New York, on a tight $14 million budget, the film got savaged by critics, who hated everything except Jim Henson's foam-rubber Turtle suits. No matter. It made a fortune—over $200 million worldwide—and spawned a franchise that would come to feature big stars like Megan Fox, Laura Linney, Will Arnett, and Tyler Perry, but none of the original Turtle actors.

Bottom line: it happens. And some voice actors take it harder than others. I reminded myself of the lesson I'd learned from Russell Johnson. Time to act like the Professor.

In the late '80s, I worked on a feature-length version of *The Jetsons*. I wasn't terribly excited about *Jetsons: The Movie*, I have to say, because we found out that the producers decided to replace the original voice of Judy Jetson, Janet Waldo.

Janet passed away in 2016 at the age of ninety-seven. But in those days she was a very active actress and very much able and willing to reprise a well-known role she helped create in a seminal animated show. The producers, however, decided to instead cast Tiffany. Yes, Tiffany, the pop singer. It wasn't Tiffany's fault. But the producers made a huge mistake, in my opinion. Not only do I think it was a crappy movie, but it completely broke Janet's heart.

The rest of us did the movie with mixed emotions and some regret. I had only minor voice roles, but it would turn out to be one of my more eventful jobs. To begin with, Mel Blanc played Mr. Spacely, Mr. Jetson's boss. Gordon Hunt, who served as the recording director on the movie, asked me if I wanted to sit next to Mel.

"Are you kidding me?" I said.

I mustered up the courage to introduce myself. I told him what a pleasure it was to meet him, how he was the voice of my childhood—all the stuff he's heard for years. Then I found myself a way to be even more obnoxious than I usually am.

"And I can't resist asking you—" I started to say.

I didn't finish the sentence before Mel said, "Eh, what's up, Doc?" in all his Bugs Bunny glory.

Now, I'm not comparing myself to Mel. But to have something like that in your career is a gift worth more than gold. So any time somebody asks me to say, "Narf!" or "Turtle power!" you bet I do it. It's the reason I do this job.

The producers of *Jetsons: The Movie* cast another legend, George O'Hanlon, the original voice of George Jetson since the 1960s. Mr. O'Hanlon was in his late seventies at the time and had already suffered a stroke that robbed him of most of his sight and some of his hearing, but not of his ability to act and sound like George Jetson.

He was frail, so his wife would accompany him to the sessions. She would sit next to him, and Gordon would feed her lines, which she would tell to George. On one particular day, we Turtles happened to be borrowing the Hanna-Barbera studio when our director, Sue Blu, stopped us in the hallway. "We've got to hold on," she said. "We've got a problem."

We found out later that Mr. O'Hanlon was doing his lines as George Jetson with his beautiful wife by his side when he all of a sudden put his hand to his head, said, "I have a headache," and slumped over onto his wife. They brought him into Gordon's office until the paramedics arrived.

We found out George O'Hanlon died at the hospital. It was sad and surreal. But I'll be honest: when you have to go, it might as well be while you're doing something you love.

After the *Ninja Turtles* movie came out, we put our heads down and did our work, lending our voices to the animated Turtles in the recording studio. I'm a realist about my role in the process. The power of this franchise comes from the characters—beginning, middle, and end. It's a power that transcends mere entertainment.

I discovered this in dramatic fashion when I did a series of charity hockey games with the Celebrity All-Star Hockey team, a great bunch of guys: Alex Trebek, Alan Thicke, Richard Dean Anderson, Jason Priestley, Dave Coulier—hockey playing actor-type folks, most from Canada or, like me, the upper Midwest.

This was late 1990, early 1991, the middle of the Canadian winter. Our first stop was in Edmonton for a game against the Edmonton

Old-Timers, all former NHL stars. This was my first trip with them, and I was able to join up because the charities that we played for were geared toward children, and at that time *Turtles* was really in full swing. I brought 250 *Turtles* pictures to sign. The kids lined up, and I autographed them as fast as I could. Alan Thicke and Alex Trebek came by.

"You're a machine, Rob," Thicke said. That's why I was there with these other more famous guys. Raphael was so popular I ran out of photos.

The next day, we went to Calgary and played the Calgary Flames Old-Timers up at the Saddledome. The event was for the Muscular Dystrophy Association of southern Alberta. I was told by the organizers that there were two kids who were the poster children from southern Alberta. And, moreover, they were from the same family, which is, I've come to find out, not unusual. Genetically that is not that uncommon. I couldn't even imagine it.

The two kids were a little boy and a little girl, Chad and Mandi Gozzola. Chad was the same age as my son, about five at the time. We went up for the pregame warm-up and to drop the ceremonial puck. They brought out little Chad in his motorized wheelchair to center ice. He was covered in *Turtles* stuff. I mean, he had a Turtles bandanna on, he had his Turtle pajamas, his wheelchair was covered with Turtle stickers. It was overwhelming. I skated over to him and I sort of just wrapped my arms around him. I didn't know what else to do.

I'm sure his parents had said, "Hey, Raphael's here," and he was probably thinking there's this bitchin' Turtle guy, and all of a sudden this weird knucklehead hockey player skates over.

Everybody was tapping their sticks on the ice. A couple of actor buddies, Kenny Olandt and Jerry Houser, skated over, and we posed for a photo.

We skated back to the guys, and they put their arms around me. I was weeping. That was the first time I'd really gotten to see such a profound example of how deeply children related to the Ninja Turtles. I'd been signing stuff for probably a year. But I'd never had an experience that affected me that way, where I could see just how important it was to this little boy and his family.

We played the game, and Chad's father somehow managed to

get ahold of me and said, "Hey, Mr. Paulsen, would it be okay if we brought Chad down to the locker room to meet everybody?"

I said that as far as I was concerned, it was fine. Remember, I was just a player, I was not the organizer. I said, "Of course." Chad and his daddy came down to the locker room, and everybody was all sweaty.

His dad told him, "Hey, buddy, this is Raphael."

Right away, Chad started calling me Raphael. I never told him my name was Rob. He, his father, his mother, his sisters, they all referred to me as Raphael, and I was fine with that.

I wanted to give him a souvenir but suddenly realized I was out of Turtle pictures. I had given them all out in Edmonton.

His father said, "Will you sign his wheelchair?"

I said, "I will, but I tell you what, I gotta do one better than that."

I realized that this was an impossibly important moment, one of those epiphanies where I said, *You have got to remember this.* Just like I remembered Mickey, the fan who said, "You're the best band in Flint," which got me to leave Flint. Just like I remembered the auditions that had made my career what it was. Well, this was one of those voice lessons. Because it was about the impact of my voice, and I was very cognizant of how important this responsibility was.

"You know what, Chad," I said, "you're not going to believe this, dude, but even though I'm a pretty smart Turtle in a lot of ways, I'm not the smartest Turtle. If I were Donatello, I'd have brought a lot more pictures, but I'm Raphael and I'm kinda the hothead of the bunch. But never fear, I'm smart enough to have something very special left over."

Mind you, we were in Calgary, so it was freezing. And the jacket I'd worn was my *Ninja Turtles* crew jacket, a varsity jacket with a typically wool body and leather sleeves and all that, with the Turtles and Raphael on it.

"I tell ya what, I'm smart enough to have brought one special gift, just for you, and it's this special, powerful jacket."

I pulled out a Sharpie and signed his sleeve: "To Chad, the best friend a turtle ever had. Turtle power."

I put the jacket around him on the wheelchair and gave it to him. His father just had to step away, and he started to cry, and I started to cry, and all the guys around me were saying, "Wow."

Once he left I kind of got my shit together, and one of my buddies said, "You really are the stupidest Turtle. What are you gonna do when you go outside, ya idiot?"

That night we had a dinner to celebrate Chad and his family and the Muscular Dystrophy Association of southern Alberta. The event was put together by Calgary firefighters. All these famous hockey players were there, and every one of them had kids who were Turtle fans and wanted a picture with me. As we were going to eat, Chad said, "Hey, Raphael, will you sit next to me at dinner?"

I said, "Is that okay with your dad?"

"Yeah, of course."

I sat next to Chad, and he was calling me Raphael the whole evening. His mom started to cut up his food for him because he had no use of his arms, or anything really, pretty much from the chest down.

He said, "No, no. I want Raphael to feed me."

I said, "Well, I'm a parent. I can certainly handle it."

She said, "Okay," and she took me aside. "Just make sure you cut the pieces in small chunks . . . " His swallowing function was very compromised, and he was constantly at risk of choking.

An hour into the evening, Chad said, "Hey, Raphael," then whispered in my ear. "I think I can walk."

I thought, *I really put my foot in it now. I never should have told him the jacket had special powers.*

"Oh, really?" I said.

"Yeah, I think I can walk. This jacket is really powerful."

"Well, you know, if you do that here in front of your parents and everybody, it'd be great, but it'd really freak everybody out. Do you know what that means?"

And he said, "Yeah."

"So, if you're gonna pull that, I dunno that this is the best time to do it. That's something you should share with your mom and dad and sister, in private. Talk to them about it."

I was kind of walking back, because remember, I didn't say, "You'll be able to walk, you'll be able to fly, you know, Jesus is healing you, you're going to get up outta that chair." I just said it was a special jacket that would give him Turtle power.

Stranger things have happened. But I didn't want us to be in the position of a devastated Chad saying, "Raphael told me I could walk and I can't!"

All of a sudden, my mind went to all of the horrible things I could've done just by trying to do the right thing.

"Now, you know," I told him, "power comes in many different ways, my friend. It's not only about walking. It's about having a sense of humor, it's about being kind to other people, it's about understanding them when maybe they're not so kind to you. Because you're a very special young man, Chad. And, I think you know that."

He said, "Oh, I know. People tell me that all the time."

"Well, it's true. So, the power that you get from this jacket will kind of just enhance your already special power. Does that make sense?"

I remember this so clearly, because I was so worried about breaking his heart. He said, "Yeah, yeah."

I said, "So, why don't you save walking for a time that's different, with your doctors, with your mom and dad."

"Okay, Raphael," he said, "I'll do that."

***

Turtles had a glorious run of 170 episodes from 1987 to 1995. I never left that very special world, not only returning for the second iteration of the show in 2012, but doing voices for video games and other projects.

To me it shows the strength of the whole franchise that they can manipulate the look of the show and the look of the Turtles, change the voice actors, and switch between 2-D versions, live-action versions with people running around in rubber suits, and CGI versions, and the show still rocks.

And now I'm doing yet another version of the franchise, a TV show called *Rise of the Teenage Mutant Ninja Turtles*, this time working on the other side of the glass as a voice director, trying to apply everything I learned from directors like Hobby Morrison and Gordon Hunt while working with people who weren't even born when the first show came out.

This thing is thirty-five years old, and here we are.

At the time, with Chad, I thought I had dodged a big bullet. But I really was telling him the truth. Children, in particular, have an unlimited sense of what's possible—that utter lack of self-conscious-ness. Children like Chad are locked in their bodies but not really aware of it when they start thinking about being Superman or Batman or a Ninja Turtle. That's something that adults lose, sometimes because we want to, and often because we don't have a choice.

Chad totally bought that I was Raphael, regardless of the fact that I was a thirty-four-year-old guy from California. This little green char-acter reinforced the powers he already had and bolstered them with his imagination. That is the essence of these heroes in a half shell.

CHAPTER SEVEN

Zany to the Max

The late 1980s and early 1990s were an exciting time to be in the cartoon biz, a period that would come to be called the animation renaissance, when studios were revamping their animation departments after a long, slow decline in the late '70s and early '80s. It was a time of energy and creativity not seen since the cartoon glory days of the 1930s and '40s. Audiences flocked to the art form on the big and small screens.

Disney's newly reconfigured animation unit put out *The Rescuers* in 1977 and *The Fox and the Hound* in 1981, then broadened into television. After former network executive Michael Eisner took over the studio in 1984, he drew on his television experience to start up Disney's first TV animation since the 1950s with *Disney's Adventures of the Gummi Bears*, inspired by the candies, and *DuckTales*, adapted from the Scrooge McDuck comics.

As the syndicated block of cartoons under the Disney Afternoon banner caught on with children, the Fox network countered with its own FoxKids block, turning to Warner Bros. for content. The Warner Bros. studio had largely abandoned its storied animation division, which gave us Bugs Bunny, Daffy Duck, and the rest of the Looney Tunes. But a $100 million deal with Fox brought it all roaring back. Warner Bros. supplied most of the FoxKids programming until it launched its own channel, The WB, a couple years later in 1993.

For voice actors, that meant work. When I wasn't at Hanna-Barbera, I was at Disney working on *DuckTales*, *TaleSpin*, *Goof Troop*, and *Gummi Bears*, then I'd dash down the freeway to Warner Bros. for their new shows. Among them was *Tiny Toon Adventures*, a younger version of the famous Looney Tunes cartoons, with Tress MacNeille as little Babs Bunny and Maurice LaMarche as Dizzy Devil. I played Fowlmouth, a chicken whose every other word was a swear word, beeped out in the cartoon. And I did Arnold the Pit Bull, which was just sort of Arnold Schwarzenegger—a giant Venice Beach pit bull that walked around in a tank top and a Speedo.

Andrea Romano handled casting and directing. I had become fairly close to Andrea at Hanna-Barbera because she was Gordon Hunt's assistant. Andrea got this great new gig at Warner Bros. as Kids' WB was becoming a studio priority. She would go on to become a legendary voice director of *Batman*, *Superman*, *Freakazoid!*, *Animaniacs*, and *Histeria!* She has so many Emmys she puts them in Barbie clothes.

Tiny Toons was the brainchild of Tom Ruegger, a New Jersey boy and Dartmouth grad who got his start in animation at Hanna-Barbera writing and producing *Snorks* and *Scooby-Doo* spin-offs. And the executive producer was Steven Spielberg, as part of a big new deal with Warner Bros. to use his magic touch to produce content. With Mr. Spielberg in charge, the show had a big budget and a full orchestra, just like the old days at Warner Bros.

Tiny Toons became a hit, winning a couple of Emmys, and it wasn't long before Mr. Spielberg came back with another show, with the same group of writers and Tom Ruegger as the showrunner. Tom approached me and said I'd be perfect for this show, which he described as a vaudeville-inspired variety program about three once-forgotten Warner Bros. cartoon characters living in the studio's landmark water tower.

I immediately knew this was the opportunity of a lifetime. There would be smart writing reflecting Tom's comedic genius and original songs backed by lush orchestration. This was a new show with never-before-seen characters that also had a strong connection with the classic Warner Bros. cartoons. This was my shot at being part of something with the potential to become a modern animation classic, much like the Looney Tunes I grew up with.

Tom said that normally he'd give me a job straight out, but since the show was new, and since it was part of Steven's deal, Mr. Spielberg himself was going to be making all the final decisions, including casting.

"You have to audition," Tom said.

"Sounds great," I said. "Where do I go?"

He gave me the times and location. I asked him what the show was called.

He said, *"Animaniacs."*

It was a long process. The studio opened up casting to all the agents in New York and LA, and from what I understand, they listened to six or seven hundred auditions for every character. It was done in person at a place called the Sound Castle in East Hollywood, where we had recorded another Warner Bros. show I'd worked on, *Taz-Mania.*

The producers gave me drawings of all the characters that fell under the *Animaniacs* umbrella. I was told their names were Yakko, Wakko, and Dot, two brothers and a sister with the last name of Warner. I got to pick and choose which characters I wanted to audition for. Since Dot was a girl, I read for Yakko and Wakko.

I couldn't glean much from the drawings. The characters were black-and-white and looked a little like Mickey Mouse. The names offered clues—Yakko probably talked a lot, and Wakko was probably crazy.

My cartoon voice activator went to work.

Different voices emerge in different ways. In cases like Hadji, the producers have a clear idea of what they want, and I try to follow their instructions. But more often it's an evolving process, a collaborative effort that relies as much on spontaneity and serendipity as it does on careful planning.

I don't consider myself a mimic or an impressionist, though there are elements of that in my work. I consider myself a performer. That said, I do cook up my own voices, and they come to me from everywhere. I've got a pretty long commute from the studios in Hollywood and the San Fernando Valley to my home on the eastern edge of the Valley, so I spend a lot of time alone in my car imagining and practicing new characters.

I might pick up an affect from somebody I hear in a shopping line or on TV. I try to find the little nuances. I home in on those nuances and the diphthongs and the way people drop consonants and add them or don't use the appropriate pronoun in front of a word that begins with a vowel. These are all things that help create an honest and believable character.

My brother-in-law, who's from Shelby, North Carolina, can speak in a generic American voice. He might say to me in that voice, "If you're not careful, you might break an arm." But if he's talking to his southern pals, he'll dial up the redneck accent and say, "Y'all best watch yourself, 'cause you might break a arm."

The key is "A arm." Immediately that hits the listeners' ear as something that's appropriate in the context of the character.

I also have dialects that I've been working on for a long time, because they're more difficult than others. A South African dialect is a very hard one for me to do. I listen to it, I try to do the best I can when I hear it, but it's strange, because if you're not careful, you start speaking in an Australian accent, which is different but sort of similar, too.

There are voices that are harder for me to do than others physically. On *The Fairly OddParents*, I play a character who's an alien that looks like an octopus with a clear head. His name is Mark Chang, but he talks like he's a surfer with a Malibu vibe. It's a balls-out voice that comes from deep in the throat, and I'm good for about forty minutes until the pipes give up.

Voicing characters is an art, but it's also a craft. There's a big difference between just having an aptitude for making your friends giggle and using those skills to pay your mortgage. Many people can conjure up a silly voice. I was certainly making them when I was a kid. Everybody can say, "Eh, what's up, Doc?"

The question is: Can they speak like Bugs all day long in all sorts of dramatic and comedic situations? It's the difference between saying, "Hey, hey, hey" or "Yabadabadoo," and bringing the characters to life in the context of the story.

I submit that voice actors are actors. When you think about it, Jack Nicholson has his little Nicholsonian things, and he does them all the time. Whether he says, "Hey, Mrs. Mulwray, you better watch out," or "Take the toast and hold it between your knees," it's different roles, but it's clearly him. We like Jack because he has that X factor that makes him a movie star, but he doesn't change the way he sounds all the time. He changes the way he behaves and the way he executes the character. Same with cartoon characters. If you listen carefully to Mel Blanc, Daffy and Sylvester are not that dissimilar, but they're different characters and they'd be performed differently. It's all in the acting.

The other key difference between amateurs and professionals is versatility. Many people are pretty good impressionists. Everybody does his own version of Christopher Walken because he's so affected and has those weird pauses.

But not everybody could do Chris Walken as a duck, or Chris Walken as a duck underwater. Or Chris Walken as a duck underwater falling in love with a starfish. And can you do the starfish, too? Then consider this: What if Chris Walken doesn't just express his love in words, but in song? Can you sing like Chris Walken underwater in love with a starfish?

I've had stranger requests.

Who knew when I was twelve or thirteen doing parody tunes that at sixty, the difference between earning a living and not would be the fact that not only could I sing, but sing in character. It's a key arrow in my quiver, one I reach for all the time, no more so than when I auditioned for *Animaniacs*.

The only instruction I got for *Animaniacs* was "Go for it."

As I said, the first thing I notice when trying out new voices is the physical characteristics of the character. If you look at an elephant, you know it's got a certain kind of voice. If you look at a whale, you know it's got a certain kind of voice, but when you look at Wakko, who isn't even a discernible creature, what do you even think?

His tongue was hanging out of his head a lot and he had this goofy hat on and he didn't have any pants on and his name implied that he was maybe a little bit left of center intellectually. He was the one who would bring a big mallet out of his goofy sack and pull out an anvil. He was the nutjob of the bunch. So I tried to offer my take on being a little nutty, goofy but not Goofy.

For Yakko, the producers told me that he was the big brother, the de facto leader of the three, and that he was called Yakko because he talks a lot. He was quick with a joke and quick with a smart quip and quicker with a double entendre.

So that was all written out for me, and then I could start to mess with that on my own and start to bring in my own sensibilities based on what the producers thought they wanted. I used my own voice to start out, because I had already done characters that were kind of quick-witted in my own voice. Raphael from the Turtles was a good example.

After I tried this for a while, one of the producers asked, "Do you do Groucho?"

I'm not an impressionist, but I can probably say, "Guess the magic word and win a hundred dollars" with the right vibe.

Then they asked, "Can you do Groucho on helium? And sing that way?"

So that's what I did.

The audition process went on for a long time. I'd read alone or with other actors. I'd do a session, then come back and do another one. I had six callbacks over a month and a half, and along the way I threw in other voices. One was for a secondary character named Dr. Scratchansniff, a sort of mad scientist. For him, I did my interpretation of Dr. Strangelove from my all-time favorite movie, but combined Peter Sellers with another character I love, Ludwig Von Drake, who's Donald Duck's uncle. I loved that thick German accent: Sellers as a duck.

Every time I'd go in and read, the producers would pat me on the back and say, "Attaboy, Rob." They kept telling me, "You're our guy. You can sing in character. You can do whatever we want you to do." And then they'd call me back for more.

I asked Tress MacNeille, who was going out for Dot, "So, what do you think?"

"I think I did pretty good. They seem like they really want us," she said.

We were all friends anyway, and they did keep saying, "Oh, it sounds good. Hang in there, man. We're paring it down." Trying to give us a nod and a wink. But you never know for sure. So many times a producer who truly wanted me would say, "You're my guy," and then something would happen and they'd say, "No, we're going to go with this other guy." It's the way it goes.

The more I auditioned, the more I felt this show was perfect for me. I had never felt more confident about a role in my career, so much so that I allowed for some hubris to seep in.

After one audition, I told Tom and Andrea, "You know what, you guys, if you don't hire me for this, you're making a big mistake."

I was laughing as I said it. They were laughing. But I'd never been more serious about a job in my life.

The final decision was up to Mr. Spielberg. He wanted to evaluate the auditions blindly, with no idea who was doing the voices, influenced only by what he heard. So the producers numbered audition takes instead of putting names on them.

Tress nailed the Dot voice from the beginning, and it really never was a competition. She's that good. She knew that playing cute was not about being cutesy.

Tress has this skill to take a character that could be one-dimensional and give her depth. Dot was cute, and she was willing to drop an anvil on your head. People can't ignore her, but when they start to make too big a fuss over her, she's like, "All right, I've had enough."

As for Wakko, a favorite surfaced in that force of nature named Jess Harnell. I had never worked with Jess, but it didn't take long to spot his talent. What he did with Wakko was take wacky in a whole different, surreal direction. Rather than go with the obvious, like I did, he suggested to the producers: What about the Beatles?

Being cartoon producers, who'll try anything once, I'm sure they all looked at each other and said, "Why not?"

That's the beauty of auditioning in front of folks. These days, so much of auditioning is done at a distance. You get the drawings and a character description, then record the voices and send off an MP3. This is to save money, but it comes at the cost of creativity. With an in-person audition, you can ask questions, bounce off ideas, try more things, dare to be weird. I perform better when I'm playing with another competent actor.

Jess had always done a spot-on impression of every Beatle. Each voice was completely distinct—John was different from Paul who was different from George who was different from Ringo. What Jess ended up doing for Wakko was Ringo as a baby.

And it was amazing.

For Yakko, they sent Steven ten recordings of their ten favorite versions of the character.

I later found out I was numbers two, three, four, seven, and nine.

I can only think it's because Tom Ruegger and the other producers, all of whom I'd worked with before, wanted me and worked to stack the deck in my favor. But they didn't do that until I had already proven myself. They didn't want to run the risk of Mr. Spielberg saying, "I've heard Rob a whole bunch of times. I'm kind of getting tired of him."

The producers also had all of us read for a secondary character named Pinky who would appear in short features sprinkled into *Animaniacs*. As it was described to me, Pinky and his cohort, The Brain, were two lab mice bent on world domination. They were modeled after two real-life people who were animation directors and creators in the Warner Bros. fold: Tom Minton was the physical model for The Brain, and Eddie Fitzgerald was the model for Pinky.

Peter Hastings was on Tom Ruegger's team, and he and Tom came up with *Pinky and the Brain*. It was a buddy comedy, not too different from Abbott and Costello, with a smart one (The Brain) and a dumb one (Pinky). The smart one thinks he's smart, but the dumb one always seems to have the better ideas.

Maurice LaMarche auditioned for The Brain. As a regular on *Taz-Mania* and on *Tiny Toons*, he was always part of the equation. Moe started out as a stand-up comedian who used to open for Rodney Dangerfield and was on the *Young Comedians* special in 1989. He's also a world-class impressionist and has always done a spot-on impression of Orson Welles.

They had a bunch of different people lined up for The Brain. But the second Moe opened his mouth, doing his Orson Welles impression, they said, "That's it."

It was now a question of who would be Pinky. My friend John Astin read for the part. John's a great actor, but he's the first one to tell you he's not about switching his voice around: "I do one voice and I'm confident in my ability, but the voice you get is mine."

When I auditioned, I did different stuff with my own voice, different attitudes of my own voice, impediments, no impediments, dialects, no dialects. Then I threw in the Monty Python Cockney thing.

I remember exactly where I was when I got the news about casting. It was March 1992, and I was running errands. My wife's passion was—and is—photography, landscapes primarily. I was picking up her proof sheets at a photo lab in Hollywood when my pager went off with my agent's phone number.

I found a pay phone and dialed my agent.

"Sweetie," she said, "you got it."

I kept it under control as I listened to her tell me that it was Mr. Spielberg who said, "I really like this idea of pairing Orson Welles with a wacky, nondescript, goofy British guy." He also liked the idea of Groucho on helium for Yakko. He even liked my Scratchansniff.

I hung up the phone and went back into the photo lab, calmly thanked the staff for the proofs, and returned to my car. I then screamed.

"I did it! I did it! I did it!" I shouted. I was bouncing in the driver's seat and thrusting my fists. People must have thought I was having a seizure.

I was about to embark on a wonderful journey. And I was going to do it with my friends, for Tress of course got Dot, and Moe landed The Brain. This show would change my standing in the acting community. It would also change my life.

After casting, the final major piece to the *Animaniacs* puzzle was perhaps the most inspired. Since the show featured all-new songs that had to embody the whip-smart, double entendre, wacky theme, producers couldn't just hire any writer. They needed a genius. They found it in Randy Rogel.

Randy was an unlikely cartoon writer. A West Point graduate, he'd worked as a sales manager at Procter & Gamble in Seattle but also had a love of show business. In his spare time, he ran a little local theater.

After a decade in corporate life, he pulled up stakes and moved with his family to Los Angeles to try to make it as a writer. He broke in writing for *Batman: The Animated Series*, then went out as a writer for *Animaniacs*. Tom Ruegger couldn't quite see Randy, with his military education and experience writing the dark and moody Batman, as a fit for the zany *Animaniacs*.

Then Randy came up with a song for the show. His audition tune landed him the job as both a scriptwriter and songwriter. It was to be the first song we'd record for the show.

So weeks later, after the show was cast and Randy was on board, I found myself at home in bed. My wife was watching TV while I had my headphones on, listening to Randy's piano guide track while reading the sheet music. I remember her looking at me strangely, because I blurted out, "This is unbelievable."

"What?"

"Let me sing a little bit of this."

"That's crazy," she said after hearing a few bars. "Is that like the countries?"

"Yeah," I said, "pretty much all the countries of the world, but they're rhymed."

"Yakko's World" was the first song Randy had written for *Animaniacs*, and it got him the job as the show's primary songwriter. It was one of those clever list songs the likes of which I hadn't heard in decades. It reminded me of that crazy, remarkably clever tune by Tom Lehrer about the periodic table of elements.

As I went through the song the first time, I was struck by how this bright, bouncy tune was deceptively sophisticated, something that I'd find reflected in all of Randy's writing. The countries not only rhymed, but they were geographically clumped. He starts with North and South America by and large, then he goes to Europe, then to the rest of the world.

And the song was visual. You could easily imagine Yakko singing and dancing and pointing to a world map, long before the first artist got to work. I'm just an actor and a singer, so I was in awe of the craftsmanship and creativity of this song. I realized that I was truly in the big leagues of animation.

I worked on "Yakko's World" for a few days, a week maybe, and then recorded my vocals for it at the Sound Castle. There was no orchestra. Randy wasn't even there, just Randy's piano guide track in my earphones playing the melody.

It was not an easy song. The lyrics fired off like a machine gun. The countries came fast and furious. It put me on a vocal tightrope, belting out an up-tempo tune to the melody of "The Mexican Hat Dance" that threatened at any moment to tie my tongue in knots. All while singing in Yakko's high, Marx-brother-on-helium register.

But I felt good about it as I was singing—grooving to Yakko, the countries pouring out, the beat tight and right. When we were done, everybody kind of looked at each other in the booth and said, "I think we got it."

After a stunned pause, the producer finally said, "Do you want to do another one?"

I said, "Sure."

So I did a second take in which I harmonized with myself. I just had them play it back and did one where I sang like a third above the melody. It wasn't as good as the first one. So we kept the first take. Easy peasy.

That was it. One take, goodbye, for a song I will probably still be singing when they put the last nail in my coffin. An orchestra later provided the music to go with my vocals, and the song was synched to the delightful animation that had Yakko bouncing around with a pointer stick in front of the map.

I like to think I'm good at my job. This wasn't my first musical rodeo, even on a bucking bronco of a tune like "Yakko's World." But there are a zillion Hollywood folks who could sing that song. The magic is being able to write it.

I've since done countless live shows on the road for the last couple of years with Randy, performing his music in small clubs and big concert halls for a show we call *Animaniacs Live*. "Yakko's World" is always the highlight of the show; Randy has updated it with a version that includes countries that didn't exist when he first wrote it.

People often ask me if I'm sick of singing that song. Not at all, man. It's when people don't want to hear it that I will get worried.

I'm always amazed at Randy's talent. Once during a performance at Joe's Pub in New York, when a subway rumbled beneath us and shook the venue, I stopped and said, "I'm sorry, hang on a second. That wasn't an earthquake, that was Ira Gershwin rolling over in his grave."

It's cartoon Sondheim. It is smart. It has internal rhymes. It is deeper, with several levels, like all of Randy's music. At the risk of using a double negative, his music is never not wonderful. Everybody doesn't like something, but nobody doesn't like "Yakko's World."

I recall that about six months after we recorded it—but before the cartoon aired—I was driving home from work and got a call.

"Rob Paulsen?" said a voice on the phone.

"Yeah."

"Jean MacCurdy."

The first place I went was: *Oh my God, I'm going to be fired.* Mac-Curdy was president of Warner Brothers Animation at the time. I couldn't think of any other reason she needed to reach me. It was your typical insecure actor response.

But she was just calling to tell me that they had gotten the first bits of animation of *Animaniacs* back from the artists. She couldn't believe how wonderful it was. She marveled about "Yakko's World" and how it fit together so beautifully.

I hung up and breathed a sigh of relief.

The next time we got the sense that we had something special was when we saw the orchestra: more than thirty pieces for every half-hour show, just like what Carl Stalling and Milt Franklyn used to do for all the old Warner Brothers Looney Tunes cartoons.

We were invited by the lead composer, Richard Stone, who has since unfortunately passed away, to see recording sessions whenever we wanted, and that was a remarkable thing to watch. We only laid down the vocals. Then these world-class players gave it that orchestration. Like Randy says, they can read music faster than we can read words.

The thing that was so mind-blowing was the response from the orchestra. I was treated like a pop star. "Yakko's here!" the musicians said, and they asked me to sign their sheet music. I kept looking over my shoulder, thinking, *Do they have any idea who I am?* I mean, I'm a voice actor. These guys have been studying the French horn for thirty years.

Once we started singing Randy's songs, all of us—cast, crew, producers—realized that "Yakko's World" was only the start. He was not a one-trick pony. After I did "Yakko's World," Jess Harnell did the states and the capitals, and on it went, one incredible song after another.

The scripts for the episodes were great and the jokes were funny. The stories were not geared strictly for children. They were purposely written to appeal to a broad audience. The edict from the top was to not condescend, and so every week we would look at each other with a raised eyebrow, thinking, *How the hell are they going to get this through?*

There were double entendres, hip cultural references, political references, movie references, lampooning of all kinds of sacred cows. And each double entendre got an exclamation point in the form of our jaunty tagline: "Good night, everybody!"

"We had been on these cartoon shows for three years, and they had given us a lot of freedom. Steven had given us a big budget," Tom would later tell me on my *Talkin' Toons* podcast, speaking of the first round with *Tiny Toons*. "So when that had wrapped up and that had been successful, they basically came to me and said, 'What's the next one? What's the sequel? What do we do next?' Now we had the freedom to really explore brand-new characters—Yakko, Wakko, and Dot, Pinky and the Brain, Slappy. Every sort of step along the way was perfectly laid out, because now we had this great experience with the actors, these voice actors. They were encouraged to bring more to the table. The writers were really in sync. The directors were brilliant. The music, of course, became a huge part. *Tiny Toons* had some great scores. Now we had some great songs to add to the mix, and that made a big difference."

Then people would start showing up to be guests on the show. Roddy McDowall and Cary Elwes and Olivia Hussey and Buddy Hackett. John Glover, Bernadette Peters, Dick Clark, Ed McMahon, over and over and over again. Did I mention Ernest Borgnine? It was probably after six months that I thought to myself, *This really became as big as I thought it would.*

To preview *Animaniacs* for the public, the studio went big. In July 1993, two months before it was to air, Warner Bros. reserved a huge meeting room at San Diego Comic-Con, the big kahuna of pop culture conventions. This was my first Comic-Con and, for once in my life, I was left speechless. Tens of thousands of comic book geeks and sci-fi fanatics, a brother- and sisterhood bound by a shared passion for fantasy and humor, many of them squeezing into spandex superhero costumes like shiny silver sausages. Our room was packed.

On the dais at the front of the room, I sat at a table next to the show's creative brain trust: Tom Ruegger and another writer-producer, Peter

Hastings, along with Warner's animation brass. On the big screen over our head beamed an episode that included the "Yakko's World" segment, the first time I had seen it with full orchestration.

The jokes killed, the song lyrics tickled, the animation leaped off the screen. The audience fell in love with our water tower trio, erupting in applause and showering us with questions at the Q&A that followed.

One woman in the front row, whom I can describe only as Patti LaBelle dressed as a Klingon, with a gold lamé getup and what looked like a pie tin on her head, stood and asked, "I have a question for Mr. Paulsen. That country song, that was you?"

"Yes, ma'am," I said.

"Did you improvise that song?"

I looked at everybody to my left and right. They raised their eyebrows, then chuckled.

Smart-ass that I am, I said, "Yes, I did in fact improvise the entire song. I got it on the first take. Then I improvised a song about everybody who plays major league baseball, in alphabetical order." She looked confused. I said, "I'm good, but I'm not that good."

Her question spoke to the genius of Tom and the other creators who pulled off an incredible feat with *Animaniacs*. The gags and comedy bits and music tumbled out in a loose, spontaneous fashion that belied years of meticulous work and planning by an international team. So many people ask if we improvised the whole show that Randy now jokes, "We tried that, but the animators couldn't keep up."

———

So much of the success of *Animaniacs* is due to Steven Spielberg. I had first worked for him several years earlier doing behind-the-scenes voice work on one of his films. I got into this little-known corner of the movie business when a woman called me out of the blue one day saying, "I have a loop group."

I said something dumb like, "That's wonderful. Do you do loops in the sky in planes? Are you loopy?"

"No," she said, "I got your name from somebody else who said you might be right for this job."

The loop group was made up of actors who record things like background conversations or lines of dialogue to be inserted into movies that were already shot, your voice coming from another actor's mouth, often when the actor's head is turned away or is offscreen so the effect isn't jarring. It's done if a line gets changed or the actor screws up or the director simply isn't satisfied with the original delivery. Another name for it is ADR, for automatic dialogue replacement.

One of the first times I worked on a loop group was for *Endless Love*, the 1981 forbidden teen romance story starring Brooke Shields and Martin Hewitt and featuring the screen debut, in a tiny role, of an unknown actor named Tom Cruise.

The looping session was overseen by the director, the Italian legend Franco Zeffirelli. I was a kid in my twenties and had no idea what he even looked like, but I sure knew his work. He directed, in my opinion, the definitive *Romeo and Juliet* in 1968, with Leonard Whiting and the incomparable Olivia Hussey, with whom I'd later work on *Pinky and the Brain*.

Zeffirelli had presence. Once he walked into the room, everyone knew at once who he was, Continental with a sweater thrown over his shoulder and an interpreter at his side.

All us loopers were lined up to meet the maestro. He walked up and down our group of actors, very kind to us, shaking our hands, never treating us like the B team. It was like a meeting with the pope.

After I shook his hand, he walked to the next actor, then came back to me. Through his interpreter he asked my name. I told him. Then in his heavily accented voice he asked me, "Rob, haven't we worked together?"

I said, "Gosh, Mr. Zeffirelli, not unless you directed some Jack in the Box commercials."

He looked at his interpreter, who said something in Italian, then the director burst out laughing. He pinched my cheek and said, "Thees one I like."

I couldn't tell you what I did on the film, though I can assure you it wasn't anything for the sex scenes.

That came later.

Warner Bros. brought me in for a looping session with my friend

Annie Lockhart—the daughter of June Lockhart from *Lost in Space*—who, like so many of us, you've heard without knowing it's her. (Most recently she voices the dispatcher on *Chicago Fire*.) Our task was to loop the famous scene in *Risky Business* in which Tom Cruise gets hot and heavy with Rebecca De Mornay on a subway train.

Annie and I were standing there in the old Warner Bros. Hollywood studio on Formosa, feigning smooching sounds, but it didn't sound right. I looked at Annie. "If we're going to do this, why do we just *do* this?" I said. "I promise I brushed my teeth."

She chuckled and said, "Okay."

If you listen very carefully, at the beginning of the scene, as Phil Collins sings "In the Air Tonight," you can just hear Annie and me kissing.

I've looped maybe twenty movies, so many I'm embarrassed to say I don't remember what I did on all of them, though sometimes I'll be watching a film and say, "Hey, that's me." We all made extra money looping in those days. In Tim Burton's *Ed Wood*, Vincent D'Onofrio played a young Orson Welles—but the voice belonged to my pal Maurice LaMarche.

My most memorable looping gig had to be for the 1987 *Star Wars* spoof *Spaceballs*, directed by Mel Brooks and starring Bill Pullman and John Candy. We had an incredible cast of loopers who'd go on to bigger and better things: Nancy Cartwright, veteran voice actor Corey Burton, and an up-and-coming improv genius from Groundlings named Phil Hartman.

A half dozen of us were in the ADR session, which Mel Brooks directed himself.

"Listen," he told us, "we got this thing coming up where Bill Pullman crashes on a big desert planet and we got these little people walking around and they're called the Dinks. They walk around going, 'Dink, dink, dink.'"

"There's this one Dink," Brooks continued, "who comes back later and brings water to Bill Pullman. I gotta have a name for that Dink to refer to him later in the movie."

I elbowed Phil. "I got something," I whispered, and I told him my idea.

Phil rolled his eyes, then said, "Tell him that."

"No, no, no," I protested.

"Tell Mel your idea," Phil pressed.

So I said, "Mr. Brooks."

"What's your name?" he asked.

"Rob Paulsen."

"Whataya got?"

"How about Gunga Dink?"

Phil gave me a congratulatory back slap. The other actors laughed.

Mel Brooks said, "What's your name again?"

"Rob," I said.

"Let me tell you something, Rob: wit is shit, funny is money. Who's got something else?"

I went on with the gig—we all said, "Dink, dink, dink"—but I was heartbroken. Phil tried to mollify me, saying that Mel was pissed because he didn't think of it. Years later, a friend of mine had Mel on his podcast and related this story.

Mel didn't remember the episode, but admitted that his "wit/shit" remark to me "sounds like something I would have said."

That's the closest I would ever get to Mel Brooks vouching for my comedy chops.

I would become good friends with Phil Hartman. Not long after this looping session he called me, excited, to say that he'd been cast in *Saturday Night Live*. To me, he was always terrifyingly inspirational. He would make what he did seem so effortless. He had incredible range and was absolutely fearless. He could inhabit a full-fledged character and make it his right away, a skill he honed in improv. I told him I wanted to be able to do that, too. Phil helped me realize it was not about mimicking his character process, it was about finding my own tools to be the best actor I could be.

I remember so clearly the day I found out that we had lost him. It was 1998. I was in Burbank, driving to a studio for a gig, when Tress MacNeille called me. She was close to Phil from their days together with the Groundlings.

"I don't know what's going on, but there's a bunch of police cars at Phil's house," she said. "You might want to turn on the radio."

The news reports said Phil had been shot to death by his wife, who also took her own life. I was shaken. I pulled over. I bought a cup of coffee from Western Bagel and sat in a daze. I still can't drive by that shop without it all coming back.

For the ADR work on the Spielberg movie, I went to the recording studio at Universal. The film was then called *A Boy's Life*. Mr. Spielberg came into the recording studio himself and told us more about the story. It involved an intergalactic thing, but he said no more. He showed us scenes in which the character was blacked out.

There was a sequence in which doctors tried to save the creature's life. Spielberg had cast real physicians to lend the scene an air of authenticity. They could rattle off the tricky medical jargon, but some of their delivery was a little dry.

A couple other actors and I then spent a few hours saying things like, "We're losing him!" to juice up the drama.

A Boy's Life wound up being called *E.T. the Extra-Terrestrial* and was a blockbuster in 1982, of course. You won't find me in the movie credits on screen. But if you call up IMDb, I'm literally the second to last person listed next to "ADR loop group (uncredited)." I still get residual checks for a buck eighty-five.

More important, I entered Steven Spielberg's universe. I did on-camera work for his show *Amazing Stories*, playing a guy who worked in the gift shop at the Alamo and then went back in time and fought with Davy Crockett. Then I got hired on Spielberg's *Tiny Toon Adventures* with many of the same voice actors on *Animaniacs*.

We had a lavish launch party for *Animaniacs* on the Warner Bros. lot at the foot of the water tower. It was September of 1993, and everybody was there—the cast, crew, writers, animators, storyboard artists, and musicians. While we were all down there for the party, Steven Spielberg shook everybody's hands and thanked us. I was there with my son, Ash, who was eight years old. Mr. Spielberg walked up to a group of us, and I'm sure that somebody said to him, "Okay, now, this is Rob Paulsen. He's Yakko."

He shook my hand. "Oh, Rob, they're so great. Pinky and Scratchansniff and Yakko. Just great work. We're so proud to have you."

He was so effusive in his praise to all of us, and before I could get it out of my mouth, he looked at my son, Ash, and he said, "Is this your boy?"

I said, "It is."

He said, "Do you think we could get a picture together?" He knew everybody wanted a picture with him, and he defused it immediately by offering. It was a small gesture but went a long way with a guy like me.

Around this time, Jess Harnell had a friend who was a really incredible airbrush artist. Jess came to work one day with a fantastic biker jacket with an *Animaniacs* logo and the three characters, Yakko, Wakko, and Dot, and the water tower and "Steven Spielberg Presents" and all that on the back of the jacket. Beautiful.

We all bought one. Ultimately we had six made. One each for Jess Harnell, Tress MacNeille, and myself, one for Tom Ruegger, the creator, one for Andrea Romano, our voice director, and one for Mr. Spielberg. We had given the jacket to Tom Ruegger and said, "Next time you see Steven at a story meeting, please give him this jacket with our compliments." A few days later, I got a phone call at home from a woman who said she worked with Steven Spielberg.

"We understand you have this jacket for him, and he was so flattered, and maybe you guys would like to come over and have lunch here at Amblin on the Universal lot?"

I thought people were screwing with me. "Yeah, thanks a lot," I said. "If you could just tell Steven I'd love to, but I'm too busy flossing my bowling ball next Tuesday."

She chuckled. "Yeah, well that happens all the time," she said. "No, this really is his office and he really was very touched by your collective offer. Do you really want to come over and have lunch and spend an hour with Steven and give him the jacket and talk about the show?"

"Absolutely," I said.

A few days later Tress, Jess, and I walked in to the Amblin offices at Universal Studios. Mr. Spielberg was a little bit late. As he came out to meet us, Tress's eyes lit up.

"Hi, Tress," he said.

"Hi, Steven," she said.

I thought, *I'm friends with somebody on a first-name basis with Steven Spielberg.*

As Mr. Spielberg brought us into the meeting room for a catered lunch, he instructed his assistant, to "hold his calls," just like important guys do in the movies, and we didn't get one interruption for the whole hour with him.

I had worked for Mr. Spielberg on *E.T.* and *Tiny Toons* and *Amazing Stories*, emphasis on work *for*—an employee, no different from thousands of others. I had never been granted this kind of face time, for Mr. Spielberg sits atop all others in my business. One phone call from him can make anything happen in Hollywood: a movie, a series, a video game. We were journeymen actors getting the Hollywood equivalent of a papal audience.

He asked us a bunch of questions about what we thought of the show and any ideas we had, took some pictures, and we gave him the jacket.

Afterward, I called my parents right away: "You are not gonna believe what I just did."

Now I know what some of you may be thinking: I'm heaping praise on the most powerful man in Hollywood, and one who for decades has been my boss. Real brave.

But I've found that there are very few people who have reached that level of success and have his class. He serves as a wonderful example of how to behave if you're fortunate enough to cultivate some sort of power and celebrity—how to walk through your life and be able to make people feel as though they are every bit as important to you as you are to them, and that's a big deal, man. He could easily be like so many other assholes in their orbits. Instead, he makes it about you, not him, and I'm convinced his interest is genuine.

Twenty years later, this became dramatically apparent when Mr. Spielberg easily could have replaced his ailing Yakko.

Yeah, I'll go to bat for Steven Spielberg.

As I said, the recurring joke in *Animaniacs* was that nobody really knows what kind of creature Yakko, Wakko, and Dot are supposed to be. While nobody ever specifically said they echoed Disney's favorite rodents, the similarities are hard to miss. Once, this turned into an uncomfortable situation.

Somebody in the promotions department in marketing thought it'd be a great idea to put this giant sort of Macy's Thanksgiving Day Parade inflatable Yakko on the water tower. Apparently nobody told Bob Daly, who was running the Warner Bros. studio at the time with Terry Semel. The story goes that he apparently came back from lunch, and this giant balloon had been inflated.

"What the hell is Mickey Mouse doing on my water tower?" he supposedly said.

Yakko was deflated and off that tower in less than twenty-four hours. I submit if you find Jimmy Hoffa, you'll also find that Yakko.

Animaniacs first aired on Fox Kids in 1993, the right show at the right time. For both FoxKids and The WB, it was a consistent ratings winner. Two years after it debuted, the *Pinky and the Brain* segments became so popular they were spun off into their own show.

As the ratings for both shows soared, Warner Bros. sent Tress, Jess, Maurice, and me on the road, usually to visit one of the new WB stores popping up around the country. While *Teenage Mutant Ninja Turtles* gave me a taste of the power of animation, it was *Animaniacs* that proved just how deeply this new generation of cartoons had penetrated the American psyche.

We had become mini-celebrities. Since we did a cartoon, many of our fans were mini, too. Moe and I once did a *Pinky and the Brain* autograph signing at a Warner Bros. studio store. It was a Sunday morning, just after church. One family came up to us with two little boys, all dressed up in their Sunday "go to church" clothes, suits and ties. They clearly had spent quite a while outside to meet us, and the wait had taken a toll on the youngsters.

I could tell that this little fellow was looking unwell, and his mom kind of fanned him, so I thought we'd better get this show on the road. We had all our pictures out and were ready to rock and roll.

"Look, it's Pinky and the Brain," the mom said to one of the boys.

I stuck my hand down and said, "Hello, what is your name?"

He answered by throwing up. I mean, from deep Down South throwing up. He threw up all over me, the pictures, everything.

The mother was absolutely mortified.

"It's okay, it's okay," I said. "I have a child. I know what projectile vomiting is all about."

I felt so bad for the little guy. I looked at him and I said, "It's quite all right. You had blueberry pancakes for breakfast, didn't you?"

"Mm-hmm," he mumbled.

They cleaned him up. He got his picture with us, minus the blue vomit. To this day I wonder if that little boy could ever watch *Pinky and the Brain* again.

As for Maurice and me, this was one of countless bonding moments. He has become one of my dearest friends, and years later, when I was getting the bejesus zapped out of my throat with radiation, Moe was the first of my animation friends at my side.

Jess I first met on *Animaniacs*. He came in as this wide-eyed kid with this ton of hair. He's a rock-and-roll singer, a great studio singer, and *Animaniacs* was the first cartoon show he'd gotten. He got a kick out of it and channeled the fruits of his success in a way that only Jess could. He too has become a close friend, and as much a character in real life as any of the roles he's voiced.

As an example, when Tress, Jess, Randy Rogel, and I were preparing for an *Animaniacs Live!* show years later, we went to Randy's house to rehearse. We were warming up with the piano when Jess called me. I figured he'd be late, because it's not unusual for him to be a little bit late. He said, "Robby, Robby, Robby, it's Jess."

"Hey, yeah, buddy. I recognize the number. You okay?"

He goes, "Yeah, I'm gonna be a little bit late. Dude, I'm so sorry. I'm stuck in an elevator."

I asked Jess where he was.

He said, "In my house." Jess had a three-story home with a toy room and a video room.

Only Jess would have an elevator in his own home.

Of all the characters I've done, Pinky holds a special place in my heart. He has not only charmed audiences of both kids and adults, but he so impressed the television community that he helped me earn three Emmy nominations in a row.

Here I have to clarify. There are Emmys and then there are Emmys. My friend Maurice has won two prime-time Emmys, in 2011 and

2012, for outstanding voice-over performance for a variety of characters on *Futurama*. These are the Emmys most people think about, the ones for shows like *Game of Thrones* and *Modern Family* that air after 7:00 p.m.

For a time there, Moe and I were eligible for a prime-time Emmy for *Pinky and the Brain*. The network bumped us to 7:00 p.m. on Sunday nights. Unfortunately that put us up against the CBS juggernaut *60 Minutes*, which had dominated the ratings in that time slot for about a thousand years. It was a death spot, and we quickly died.

Pinky and the Brain returned to its rightful afternoon slot and did just fine, collecting all kinds of trophies at the daytime Emmys, the ones that honor shows that air during the day, like soap operas, talk shows, game shows, and children's programming.

In May of 1997, I was up for my first daytime Emmy for playing Pinky. They threw a huge awards show at Radio City Music Hall, with Susan Lucci and Regis Philbin hosting. Fred Rogers got a lifetime achievement award for Mr. Rogers.

Although I didn't stand a chance against the all-star nominees— Louie Anderson for *Life with Louie*, Lily Tomlin for *The Magic School Bus*, Dennis Franz for *Mighty Ducks*, and Rita Moreno for *Where on Earth Is Carmen Sandiego?*—this was a big deal for me and my family. I brought Parrish, Ash, and, at Parrish's insistence, my mother, Lee.

Of course nobody knew who the hell I was. But Mom got a big kick out of it, and so did I. From the first time she introduced "Robin Paulsen and his neckitar" in the living room, my mother was always my biggest fan. She would have been impressed if my career had ended with the Jack in the Box commercial. I wanted to give her a gift nobody else could.

We drove all of eight blocks in a limo then walked the red carpet, where the photographers of course had no idea who the hell any of us were.

When I was very young, my mom used to say, "If your horn is worth blowing, somebody will blow it for you." So she turned to the photographers and said, "My son is here because he was nominated for an Emmy. Do you watch *Animaniacs*?" Then, to me: "Do the voice, Rob."

After I did a little Pinky, my mom said, "That's my son."

Louie won the Emmy, but no matter. It was worth it just to see my sweet mom so happy in her beautiful dress, accompanying her goofy oldest child to this fancy-schmancy Emmy thing.

The next year, the show moved to Los Angeles, and I scored another nomination for *Pinky and the Brain*. Once again, Anderson took the prize. I made it a hat trick in 1999. This time, it was now or never. Season four of *Pinky* was wrapping up, and we hadn't recorded anything new. The same for *Animaniacs*. Although no official announcement was made, it looked like it was over. The actors had already begun working on other shows.

This had been a difficult year for my wife. She was diagnosed with breast cancer in January of 1999, and three months later her father died. The radiation treatments had knocked her for a loop, and to this day she doesn't feel 100 percent. By the time of the Emmys in May, she was cancer-free but still on the mend from the treatments.

So with the Emmys bouncing back to New York, we turned it into a celebration of my wife's health. The ceremony was everything we had hoped for. My wife looked like a zillion dollars in her beautiful Gilles Savard gown, and my boy and I cleaned up pretty good, too. After two years of rentals, I bought my first tux. Warner Bros. went all out, sending a big contingent and planning an after-show bash at the swanky 21 Club.

After the red carpet, I sat with my wife and son and the entire WB contingent from Los Angeles. Our category came up, and despite my two previous losses, I was still full of nerves. They have a camera right there in your face. The presenters were Whoopi Goldberg from *The View* and Tom Bergeron from *America's Funniest Home Videos*. They announced the nominees: Louie Anderson again, Dom DeLuise and Ernest Borgnine from *All Dogs Go to Heaven: The Series*, Jeffrey Tambor from *The Lionhearts*, and yours truly.

I again wasn't feeling good about my chances. But the fact that it was four big names and some guy from Michigan made this all the more important to me. I felt like I was representing the voice acting community who, by and large, were still relatively anonymous.

A lot of what came next was a blur. I know I heard my name. I know I freaked out and dashed up to the stage. I remember looking out at the audience and spotting Rosie O'Donnell, Barbara Walters, and Susan Lucci, who had made news that year by breaking her epic losing streak, winning her first Emmy in nineteen nominations for *All My Children*.

"Wow," I said, "I'm the only person here I don't recognize."

I remember thanking my wife and my son and Mr. Spielberg and Tom Ruegger and Andrea Romano and Jean MacCurdy and everybody else at Warner Bros.

I remember looking in the crowd and seeing in the third or fourth row the hockey star Wayne Gretzky and his wife, Janet. Wayne was finishing his career with the New York Rangers, and they attended the ceremony because they were both big soap opera fans.

I remember saying, "And Wayne Gretzky, you're not gonna believe this, but I was in your basement two weeks ago."

The audience kind of chuckled like, "Who is this man and why's he making an ass of himself?"

As fried as my synapses were, I was speaking the truth. I had been to his house.

I had been invited to a children's charity golf tournament somewhere in southern Ontario. I played some golf, signed some autographs, and gave the keynote speech. The morning they picked me up at my hotel to go to the event, I was told we had to make one stop in Brantford, which is a small town in Ontario, to pick up another fellow who was going to join us. We pulled into a little home, and they told me to go to the door and get the guy. His name was Walter.

I knocked, and Walter Gretzky answered.

"You must be Rob. I've heard all about you. I understand you're a hockey player," he said.

"Yeah," I stammered, "I'm a hockey player."

Mr. Gretzky is almost as famous as his son in hockey circles. I was transfixed, humbled, and nervous just to be there.

He said, "How about coming downstairs and having a look in the basement? We've got all of Wayne's stuff. It's getting ready to be shipped off to the hockey hall of fame."

He had everything, and I mean everything, down to the first tooth that got knocked out of Wayne's mouth, the first stick Wayne ever used, the first Wheaties box he was ever on, the first Campbell's soup can he graced.

I must have spent a half hour down there. It was miraculous. It was just too cool to miss, too cool to not mention at the Emmys. To this day I'm sure Wayne Gretzky wonders just what the hell I was talking about.

At the Emmys, there's a big clock with a minute timer in the back of the theater showing the time you get to say your thank-yous. I looked over to stage left, and Dick Clark, the producer of the show, was in the wings pointing to his watch and doing that circling-the-finger motion that means "Wrap this up."

I got done, or thought I was done, but as I walked off the stage, I stopped dead in my tracks. I looked at Whoopi Goldberg and said, "Holy shit, I didn't thank Maurice."

I mean, it's not called *The Pinky Show*.

She said, "You can't go back out there now, honey."

My first task, once I got down to the bowels of Madison Square Garden, was to find a pay phone so I could make a call to Maurice to let him know: a) that I won, b) that I forgot to thank him on television, and c) how sorry I was. He didn't answer, so I left a message, then went back upstairs feeling terrible. (We later embraced when I got back to LA. He's still including me in his plans for world domination, last I checked.)

I was standing backstage, waiting to go in to speak to the press about my little Emmy, when I felt a tap on my shoulder. I turned around and it was Fred Rogers. The day was becoming more surreal by the minute. I believe he probably did this to everybody, but he took my hand with two of his. He looked me right in the eye, and he said, "Young man"—I was forty-three at the time—"congratulations. Your parents must be so proud of you."

To this day it chokes me up thinking about it. All I could say was, "Thank you so much, Mr. Rogers. I don't know how to thank you. This means so much to me."

He remarked about how important children's television was and said I conducted myself beautifully onstage. In an instant I recognized what it was about him that made him so special. He exuded class, gentleness, a grace that was palpable. It was like I had been blessed by the pope. He was a very special human and my one- or two-minute exchange with him was worth a lifetime of joy and inspiration. Incredible.

Another individual who came up to me afterward and was just delightful was my fellow nominee Louie Anderson. "I never had the pleasure of meeting you, but I want to congratulate you," he said. "You're the only one that really should win one of these goddamned things."

I never went back to my seat. Somewhere out there might be a guy who made a few bucks as a Rob Paulsen seat filler, you got me. My wife and son and I, all decked out in our formal wear, grabbed a cab for my brother Mike's house. He lived close by in Hell's Kitchen with his then partner, now husband, Jim.

He answered the door, and I could see the awards were still playing on TV. I held up my Emmy, and my brother and brother-in-law went nuts. After we left my brother's place, we went to 21.

The next day, I walked through JFK airport with my wife and son and, so help me, my Emmy. I couldn't help myself. We got on the plane and the flight attendant said over the speaker, "We have an Emmy winner here, Rob Paulsen," and everybody applauded.

Rightly or wrongly, awards represent credibility in Hollywood. I'm now an Emmy-winning actor. On the other side of the coin: I won an Emmy for a cartoon show.

I don't get better tables at restaurants. My price didn't go up. I didn't all of a sudden start commanding 300 percent more in salary. I even had producers whom I met after I won the Emmy, six or seven months later, say, "Hey, congratulations. Gosh, I hope we get to work together again. I hope we can afford you," and they'd kind of chuckle.

"Are you kidding me?" I'd say. "Call me."

The statue holds a special place in my home. It makes for a good conversation piece, like when somebody comes over to fix your furnace and they walk through the house and say, "Wow, is that an Emmy?"

I say, "Yes, it is," and I tell them what I won it for.

Then their face drops. "Oh, a daytime Emmy."

I realize that a daytime Emmy and five bucks will get you a grande Frappuccino at Starbucks.

But this Emmy is my Emmy. And I'm going to keep it.

CHAPTER EIGHT

Pinky Needs Work

At those same 1999 Emmy awards, *Pinky and the Brain* won for outstanding animated program, its first show Emmy, and *Animaniacs* picked up an award for music direction and composition, the eighth Emmy for the show, to go with a prestigious Peabody.

It turned out to be a glorious send-off. I'm not going to presume to know the real reasons why *Animaniacs* and *Pinky and the Brain* got the ax. The studios don't consult with the voice actors when they green-light a show, and they certainly don't consult with us when they pull the plug. I've heard many theories, from slipping ratings to—my favorite—the shows appealed too much to adults, and I'll be honest, I can't confirm any of them.

It's always tough when a show ends, but none of us went into mourning. By all indicators, it was a hell of a run. We did ninety-nine episodes of *Animaniacs* and sixty-five episodes of *Pinky and the Brain*. That's unusual for any show not called *Ninja Turtles* or *The Simpsons*. I just felt fortunate to be a part of it.

Besides, there was no time to grieve. I was busier than ever. Even as *Animaniacs* and *Pinky and the Brain* were chugging along, I worked for other shows. Among them was the animated version of the hit comedy *The Mask*. I voiced the lead character, Stanley Ipkiss, who would put on the mask and transform into different characters germane to the situation: a pirate, short-order cook, cowboy, astronaut, gold miner, fur trapper.

I assume the producers hired me for the cartoon because they couldn't afford Jim Carrey, who was Ipkiss in the live-action version. But he very much was a presence in the studio. A half a dozen times during the first recording sessions, the producer would say, "Remember in the movie, when Jim does it this way"—fill in the blank. "Let's do it like that."

I got that I was merely a less expensive version of Jim, and I tried to give the producers exactly what I thought they wanted. But I'm an actor, not an impressionist. Plus, the movie was only two hours. We had thirteen episodes planned; that's more than six hours of animation. *Soon this character should be as much me as Jim*, I thought. Slowly I began extrapolating and expanding. They kept wanting more of what they thought Jim would do.

I was getting frustrated. I didn't know how to make these people happy. One day, I complained to Tim Curry, who played the character called Pretorius.

"I'm a little confused," I said. "I'm never going to be Jim Carrey, and I thought they knew that when they hired me."

He suggested I tell the producers what I told him. This meant, of course, I could lose the gig. Another uppity actor. I decided it was worth the risk. It was still early in the production. If they wanted to put more money in the meter on this show, it was time to think about another Stanley. It wouldn't be the first time I'd been replaced, and it wouldn't be the last.

I stifled any impulse to say this in a smart-ass way and said as calmly as possible that they weren't always going to get Jim Carrey. They might start getting a little more Rob Paulsen. It was a professional discussion about the creative process, and I'm happy to report that after that everything went well.

So well, in fact, that they even expanded my role in the show. Originally, the very cool theme song was to be sung by the great Jack Sheldon of "Conjunction Junction" fame. But the head of children's programming at CBS said, "You're the Mask, you're Stanley Ipkiss, why don't you sing it?" The theme is this killer, up-tempo, big band tune that really swings. I was thrilled to do it, and to this day I think it's one of the best things I've ever done.

The work piled up. I voiced several characters for *Johnny Bravo*, a guy named Travis Lum for *Ozzy & Drix*, characters known as Boomer and Brick for *The Powerpuff Girls*, Mac Gopher for *Duck Dodgers*, Malsquando for *Dave the Barbarian*.

Then I got to meet a little guy who, I'll be honest, has become one of my best friends.

John Davis and Steve Oedekerk had asked me to read for an animated feature movie about a boy and his sweet chubby pal. The star, Jimmy Neutron, is a precocious ten-year-old with a giant Bob's Big Boy do. He lives with his parents in a town called Retroville and has a robot dog he created called Goddard, named after rocket scientist Robert Goddard. Jimmy's got two best friends, Sheen Estevez and Carl Wheezer, a plump kid who needs an inhaler and is painfully shy but always wants to be part of Jimmy's posse.

The producers asked if I had anything for Carl.

"Oh, I might have something here," I said.

In the early '90s, I did a show called *Goof Troop* for Disney. If you recall in the Disney cartoons of yesteryear, Goofy had a nemesis/neighbor named Pete, this bellicose, gruff kind of guy. In the new *Goof Troop*, Jim Cummings played Pete, and I played Pete Jr., better known as P.J. After seventy-eight episodes over two seasons, *Goof Troop* ended. But I kept playing around with that voice. One of the things I talk about a lot in personal appearances and acting workshops is how to take existing stuff or bad impressions, or even good impressions, and tweak them into a brand-new character.

That's how Carl Wheezer was born.

I took Pete Jr., softened the voice and gave him a lazy *L*, like Tom Brokaw, so that he has trouble saying names like "Larry the llama."

I landed the gig and worked alongside a good friend, Debi Derryberry, who did Jimmy. Yep, Jimmy Neutron, like Bart Simpson, is voiced by a woman.

I love Carl He is completely benign. Every girl loves Carl because he's their friend. I admit, I drew a lot from my own high school experience. I was never a particularly handsome fellow, and the girls would be like, "Oh Rob, you're just so great. I'm so glad we're friends." That was my lot until I had the good fortune of meeting my wife. Carl is the ultimate permutation of that in my life.

He's cute, he's funny and doesn't know he's funny, and just sweet. Also, when he falls down, he says things like, "Ow, my scapula." I think that's funny. *Scapula* is one of those words that makes me smile.

Jimmy Neutron: Boy Genius marked my first major motion picture for which I was hired to be a main cast member. Although it did have a couple of celebrities—Martin Short and Patrick Stewart were both in it playing bad guys—they weren't in the primary cast. Released in 2001, *Jimmy Neutron: Boy Genius* made over $80 million on a $30 million budget and was nominated for an Academy Award the first year animated films had their own category. It lost out to the original *Shrek*. The movie spawned several TV series and video games, blessing me with more opportunities to voice a beloved character.

Carl has paid for most of my cars—not my house, but most of my cars. Thank you, Carl. "You're welcome, Rob."

I became fast friends with Jimmy Neutron's cocreator, John Davis. I went to Dallas, primarily to visit the folks at DNA Productions, which did the animation for the *Jimmy Neutron* movie and the TV show. I wanted to see how talented these kids were.

While I was there, John said, "I got a script I think Tom Hanks wants to make." I guess Tom Hanks had the rights to it and took it to Warner Bros. John Davis was involved because of his experience with *Jimmy Neutron*.

The film was *The Ant Bully*, and I had a nice little role as a talking beetle. The primary cast was loaded: Paul Giamatti, Meryl Streep, Nic Cage, Julia Roberts.

I thought it was a charming enough movie. It was certainly not meant to be *The Brothers Karamazov*. The script was, I guess, okay-ish, but I presume the idea was that with all those movie stars, we'd get butts in the seats. Despite a ton of talent with a pile of Oscars, it tanked, grossing $28 million on a budget of $50 million. Certainly coming after *A Bug's Life* and *Antz* didn't help. America had clearly tired of talking insects.

Jimmy Neutron, which didn't have big stars in the leads, is to this day one of the shows that people remark about in terms of what a wonderful impact it made on them, and now on their own children. *The Ant Bully*, on the other hand, is one of those, "Oh, yeah, I think I remember that. I think I saw it on DVD or something. You were in that?"

There you go. You just never know.

Don't get me wrong. I'm not one of those voice actors who gets upset when celebrities come in and get major animated roles. I'm a capitalist. If a studio wants to shell out a half-million bucks and get Brad Pitt to be a talking monkey, great. I certainly get why celebrities want to do it. They come into the studio, have a great time in their pajamas, and go home.

I'm just saying, without the script and endearing characters, you got bupkis.

I didn't realize it yet, but the disappointment with *The Ant Bully* in 2006 turned out to be a warning sign. I had been on a roll in recent years, landing successful series, creating memorable characters. But along the way, I always reminded younger actors to be ever vigilant of the precarious plight of the business of acting. Once at a workshop, an acting student told me, "I can't wait until I'm in your league." I offered fake modesty, which only encouraged her. She noted that I'd won an Emmy, and I'd done this and I'd done that. "Everybody knows your work."

Then I leveled with her. "Let me tell you something: after I have this chat with you, I'm going to audition for the voice of a talking ice cream cone."

These days, I get my share of work without having to read for somebody. But the fact is, when you're not a major celebrity talent—and I am not, by any stretch of the imagination, a major celebrity talent—you still have to hustle. You still have to prove yourself, over and over. It doesn't matter how established you are in Hollywood or what kind of ratings your shows got or how much one of your movies made or how many Emmys line your shelves.

I would venture to say that I've probably booked three or four hundred jobs from auditions. If I were a baseball player, a .333 lifetime batting average would get me into the hall of fame. In show business, it means the work to get work never stops.

By late 2009, I began one of those inevitable slumps I warned other actors about. I auditioned, then nothing. I auditioned—again, nothing. Auditioned, and boom: I got three in a row, then I got nothing again.

Then nothing, nothing, nothing, and more nothing.

At first, I attributed this to how the shows had changed the audition process. More auditions were held remotely, either in an agent's office or at home, with no other actors. Mine were pretty much always at home. Disney or Universal would now send out the word: "Here's this critter, here's what he looks like, here's the way this character interacts with other folks, here are some lines. Give us your best shot. We'd like four takes."

I get why they do it. It's less expensive. You can get five hundred auditions without having to hire a casting service. But at the time, I didn't want to accept the fact that things were headed the way of the buffalo vis-à-vis in-person auditions.

I didn't like the new system at all. I didn't have that benefit of asking questions or of seeing how people would respond and react: "Hey, we never thought about that. Sure, why don't you try it?" I got a lot of work earlier in my career because I thought outside the parameters of what was given to me at an in-person audition. I didn't have that leg up anymore. Consequently, my booking ratio had fallen precipitously.

Meanwhile, I continued to buy expensive cars. Around this time it was an Aston Martin Vantage. I was a big James Bond fan, and I just had to scratch that itch. I'm driving in this fancy car to play golf for the fourth day in a row...and I'm not working that week. And I had nothing the next week.

At the end of 2009, my wife wanted to do a remodel on the home we had bought in 1989. "Sure, no problem," I said, and off I went to my Happy Place: *It will pick up. It always has.* My wife recruited two people to sketch out the plans. It wasn't a teardown, just a remodel, and not even a big one. Work was set to begin in early 2010, but I was down to one regular gig.

It was a steady job doing a character I'd helped create. Back in 2003, I had been working with an ad agency director on radio ads for Honda. As we were recording in a studio in Santa Monica, he said, "I'm thinking about pitching an animated little two-dimensional guy to Honda for their year-end clearance sale." He asked if I would mind laying down some demo tracks. He said he couldn't pay me, but this could help him get the commercial deal. Unspoken was that it could also help me land the voice gig later on.

He handed me some copy and said, "The only problem is we don't have a real tagline."

"What's this guy called?" I asked.

"His name's Mr. Opportunity."

It hit me in an instant. I read his copy about the 2004 Honda clearance, and then I tapped on the microphone. "You hear that?" I ad-libbed. "That's me knocking. I only knock once."

The director beamed. "Oh my God, Rob, that was great."

About a week later, the director called me. "Robby, I think you just paid for your kid's college."

For the next seven years, Honda used me and my opportunity-knocking tagline. The ads were sweet and silly. One even had my animated alter ego trying out his awkward white-guy dance moves in a club to techno music. He called his dance "The Knock."

But in 2010, Honda called and said, "We're done with that campaign." They had a new guy, Patrick Warburton, who would be on camera instead of animated.

For the first time since I was cleaning sink traps at the Esplanade apartments, I was an unemployed actor.

As I look back now, this was a slow-moving disaster. My career had been slipping for about six months, the checks getting increasingly smaller, while the lifestyle remained the same. The longer this went on, the more anxious I became. I remember having panic attacks. I would be taking a shower and find myself, for lack of a better term, just gagging, like I couldn't get my breath. It got to the point where I don't think I slept more than maybe two hours in a row each night, my mind spinning.

I worried about money, the money we didn't have at the time and the money we might never have.

Now, I want to pause right here and make something very clear. True, I was not working. But I was not broke. Nobody was going to haul me to debtor's prison any time soon. Cartoons had been very good to me. We had money in the bank, retirement accounts, health insurance. We had a vacation home. Did I mention the Aston Martin?

Yes, if the work slump continued, we would probably have to scale back. I might have to drive a Honda.

But the real problem, for me, went far deeper than dollars and cents.

I didn't just fear I'd hit a nasty slump. I feared I had hit a wall. A big, thick, brick wall—*splat*, like Wile E. Coyote. I feared I was done, over, kaput. Toontown had a room waiting for me in the Washed-Up Turtles Home, and all I could think of were those most dreaded words in Hollywood.

You'll. Never. Work. In. This. Town. Again.

And I had no solution. I couldn't figure out how to get the phone to ring. The only time I'd been in this position before was when I was first starting out in Hollywood. Back then, I didn't know how to get back on track, because I'd never been on track to begin with. Now I was a so-called animation star. I had an Emmy. Steven Spielberg had served me lunch in his office. I thought I was past all this.

Or maybe, said an unhelpful voice in my head, *maybe I was fooling myself*. Maybe I was never the hotshot I thought I was, but instead had been skating by all these years on charm and luck through a career that was as fleeting and fake as a Saturday morning cartoon.

I could hear that little voice telling me that I was finally busted. A little voice that sounded suspiciously like my father's. At the time, he was in the later stages of Alzheimer's (my mother had died after a long illness three years earlier). I couldn't discuss any of this with him if I wanted to. Even if I could, he had his stock criticisms, and I had my stock comebacks. I knew his position all too well.

Maybe my father was right all along, insisted the little voice. Performers often wrestle with the fear that what we do doesn't really matter, that our vocation isn't real in the conventional sense. It leaves us feeling insecure and craving validation. That's why we cry when we win a People's Choice Award (still waiting).

I should have talked to my wife. I should have been honest with her about what was going on.

To this day, I'm awful at delivering bad news. I never want to make anybody unhappy. I'm an entertainer, a people pleaser. The sun will come out tomorrow, as the song goes. In an effort to keep that sun shining, I tried the old tricks: evade and improvise. So desperate was I to avoid making my wife disappointed in me that I lied. That's the bottom line. I didn't only deflect. I was given every opportunity to say that we couldn't afford this house project right now, and I didn't. For months I kept up the ruse that we were flush with money.

This time, though, I wasn't going to be able to turn that D into a B. With the workers ready to start knocking out drywall, I had no choice but to fess up. We had to pull the plug on the remodel.

Then I checked into a residential motel. I couldn't face my wife. I had no explanations. I felt ashamed.

I spent two weeks there, though it felt like an eternity. I was fifty-four years old, waking up in a hotel room a couple of miles from my home, separated from my family and everything I found comfortable and familiar, with no work booked, driving a car I couldn't afford.

I didn't feel confident that things would be okay. I was in such despair that I was even unable to see the struggles of others. I was becoming more self-centered the longer this went on. So I talked to my friend Maurice—The Brain, as wise as ever. I told him the business was changing, that I was an old dog, that maybe I was done and I didn't want to be.

Moe said the usual stuff: "We all go through this. We're all a little on the edge. In this business, we're all a little eccentric." He said I was probably the most normal person he knew. He said I'd find a way back.

"Moe," I said, "I honestly don't know if I will. I'm absolutely lost."

My other friends and agents were there for me, too, when I told them I couldn't get any work.

"Are you kidding me?" they said. "You're Rob Paulsen."

Yeah, so.

"Dude, it's just really slow," others would say, and I could see the thought balloon: "Oh, cry me a river. Things are slow for *you*?" Meaning, everything is relative. What's slow for Rob is a bonanza for other actors who are lucky to work three times a year in between waiting tables. Suck it up. I even went to my doctor, who chuckled and said, "Welcome to midlife."

It was embarrassing for me to talk about. I lost twelve pounds. I couldn't eat. I'm not, by nature, a brooding guy. I like to think people enjoy working with me. It wasn't normal for me to be anxious and sad and worried. It got a hold of me, and I hated it.

When you make your living as adorable talking animals, this attitude can be problematic. Nobody wants to hire a depressed squirrel.

And the trouble was, no matter how good an actor I thought I was, I couldn't hide the despair. Hollywood may have changed some since I started out, but it could still smell fear and desperation. If I auditioned thinking I really needed that job, I was dead.

It was hard for me to get to a place where I could be honest about this, even with my agent. I remember having a really important lunch with her when Parrish and I were separated.

"This is killing me," I said. "I don't know what to do."

Not being ready to retire is not uncommon. I could give you a long list of actor colleagues who had long since called it quits by their mid-fifties. I couldn't admit how much that hurt—how much it hurt my pride to be honest with myself that it might be time to retire.

Wouldn't you know, it was Yakko who bailed me out, along with some very, very dear friends. Steve and Julie Bernstein, the Emmy-winning composers who worked with me on *Animaniacs*, phoned me while I was still at the residential hotel.

"We got a call from someone asking if we knew Rob Paulsen," they said.

In my dark and self-centered little place, I couldn't imagine anyone wanting to be associated with me. The Bernsteins explained they were working with the Cleveland Youth Symphony, doing concerts and seminars on writing music for cartoons. A colleague, the conductor of the Kentucky Symphony Orchestra, had reached out to them. His kids were big cartoon fans, and he'd noticed that somebody named Rob Paulsen had done the voices of some of his kids' favorite characters. He wondered if I would do an evening of *Animaniacs* music.

I had long wanted to perform live again, just like in the old days of fronting Sass in Michigan. But until now, I just hadn't had the time.

I told them I was happy to do it. At least those were the words I used. But I didn't feel it. Even as I said it, my voice was quivering. I hoped they didn't notice.

What I was really thinking was: *There's no way I can do this. I am absolutely a shadow of myself.* The day before, I had been driving around aimlessly. I couldn't even find the hotel where I was staying.

Regardless, I knew I couldn't turn down the work—any work. The show was set for May, just weeks away. The deadline freaked me out. I had to find a way to unfreak.

It was an evening of cartoon music conducted by J. R. Cassidy in a lovely theater on the waterfront of the Ohio River, which separates northern Kentucky and southern Ohio. Julie and Steve were there, discussing how a cartoon is scored and orchestrated, with the music from the maestro's orchestra timed perfectly to clips of animation.

I arrived in Kentucky a nervous wreck. It was a full house, and not one that appeared to be overly familiar with cartoons. Most of the audience members were older season ticket holders who, I presumed, would not have watched *Animaniacs*. There was also a reporter there from the *Cincinnati Enquirer*.

As I took the stage, my stomach churned and my mouth turned dry. This had never happened to me before; from the first time I sang with LS Phreaque, I had never experienced anything close to stage fright.

I had gone casual: jeans, untucked dress shirt, sport jacket, all of which were too big for me after losing that weight. I fiddled with my jacket, the lights went down, and a big screen over the orchestra flashed the title card: "Yakko's World. *Animaniacs*," followed by, "Featuring Rob Paulsen as Yakko." The titles noted the music was "Traditional" and the lyrics were by Randy Rogel.

As the conductor waved his baton and the timpani rumbled, I said in a deep announcer's voice, "And now, the nations of the world, brought to you by Yakko Warner."

Yakko leaped onto the screen overhead and started dancing to the beat of the live orchestra. I cracked my knuckles and jumped into the deep end: "United States, Canada, Mexico, Panama..."

I had sung "Yakko's World" countless times at conventions and other public appearances, but never with an orchestra and never synced to the animation. It was daunting and wonderful. I had never flubbed the song before, never even worried about flubbing. My nerves started to rattle and I started thinking, *What if, what if, what if? What if I got a half beat off? It would ruin the entire illusion.* Then I would mentally slap myself back to the task at hand.

I powered through the song, my emotions seesawing, desperately chasing away the fears, as the song ended with the pace at top speed: "Fiji, Australia, Sudan!"

Then, just like that, it was over. I took a breath.

The crowd whooped and whistled. As the lights came up, I shook the maestro's hand, bowed and waved, and floated off the stage.

I did two more songs that night: "Yakko's Universe" and a little ditty in which Pinky sings about cheese. But once I got through "Yakko's World," I was good.

After the show, I mingled with the audience in the lobby, meeting these lovely people who were used to seeing Mahler or Shostakovich or Mozart or Debussy or maybe the music from *The Music Man*. Folks were coming up excitedly, saying, "Oh my God, that song about all the...what is that song?"

I had crossed some sort of threshold. I was flung back in time. I was back in the Esplanade apartments again, a kid trying to make it in a tough new business. I didn't care about money or cars or home restoration projects, about agents or auditions. I just wanted to perform. I just wanted to be creative.

I felt like I had something to look forward to, to prepare for, to challenge me. There was magic in Randy's music, magic in those characters, magic in doing it live.

As I posed for photos and signed autographs, I realized that we had more than just a parlor trick here. Randy's music really is standalone interesting. It doesn't have to be etched in someone's brain from childhood in order for them to enjoy it. Randy and I needed to find some way to take this show on the road.

I remember a song from when I was a kid. It might have been on *Captain Kangaroo*—it's funny how this stuff stays with you. The song was all about facing the music. Face the music when you've got trouble, face it and you'll chase it far away. I have to say, it's a lesson I'm still trying to learn.

I returned to my home. I had those difficult conversations with my wife that I should have had so many months earlier, about honesty and fear and not always being blinded by the sunshine. Positivity is great, but even a knucklehead actor can be positive and still acknowledge the reality facing him.

I apologized, a lot. I listened and I learned. I'm still learning.

———

As for show business, if Hollywood didn't want me, I had to find a different way to be creative. I called a good friend named Mark Evanier, a very successful animation writer who's deeply involved in the annual San

Diego Comic-Con. "I've been thinking for a long time about doing a one-man show," I said. "How do I book one of the rooms at San Diego Comic-Con?"

"What kind of show do you have?"

"I don't have a show."

"What's the show going to be?"

"I don't know."

So began my career as the solo artist known as Rob. Thanks to the graciousness of the Bernsteins and the great people of Cleveland, I was determined, if somewhat clueless.

There had to be another way to ply my trade that didn't rely on recording studios, casting agents, and producers. I did research online about comedy festivals and conventions. Where would I fit in? How would I fit in?

Another dear, übertalented friend of mine, B. J. Ward, who was married to Gordon Hunt, had a successful one-woman show. She is a bona fide opera singer, and at the time she did a stand-up comedy/opera hybrid show. She would sing beautifully like Maria Callas or Beverly Sills or Joan Sutherland, and then she would do stand-up on the absurdity of so many of these operas.

It was really good. She got booked all over the world at cabarets, and she was hugely successful. I was sitting in a Starbucks at like one o'clock on a Wednesday afternoon, because I wasn't working, and I called her up. I wanted to know how I could hire myself like she did.

"Oh, honey, you can so do this," she said. "Do you have any idea? Do you know who you are?"

Whether it was true really didn't matter. It was the fact that a peer, somebody who was married to an icon in the Hollywood theater community, was encouraging me. It was nothing but love and support.

I asked her how she got started.

"Honey, Gordon put my show together," she said. I could hear her put the phone down and yell, "Gord, Rob is interested in doing a one-man show."

In the background I could hear him say, "Tell him I want to do it with him or he can't do it."

I've got to tell you, I got teary. I was already pretty raw. I was trying to figure out ways to kick myself in the ass. Here was my chance to do what I loved again. I had been feeling too much self-pity to see what was right in front of me.

"Look at the characters," B. J. said. "You can incorporate all these funny, iconic characters in a show."

With Gordon and B. J.'s input, I started to find a way out. It occurred to me that Gordon had mentored me in the beginning of my career and was mentoring me when I thought my career had ended. Asking for help and showing weakness went against my upbringing and my father's values. Later, when I spoke at his funeral, I thanked him for teaching me by example to be utterly self-sufficient. I never wanted to be a burden on anybody. I lived by the credo that if I was going to fail, it was my fault and nobody could bail me out. I was also embarrassed. I was Pinky, for God's sake, a beloved cartoon character. I was a success.

But I came to learn that the real sin is in not asking for help. And that it's never too late to ask.

What began as a discussion about doing a one-man show morphed into starting a podcast. I'd been invited as a guest on many of them. If nothing else, I figured, the Comic-Con phenomenon had proved a deep interest in my line of work. Conventions for cartoons, comic books, superhero movies, and manga had been popping up around the country. I'd been around so long that I personally knew almost everyone from whom any cartoon fan would want to hear: Bart Simpson, Homer Simpson, Goofy, Donald, Wakko and Dot, The Brain. Come on, I knew all these people.

One day, looking at my phone that wasn't ringing, I just thought, *I don't think you have to be an MIT grad to do a podcast.*

My friend Chris Pope got ahold of me and started booking me at this thing called Dragon Con, a big convention in Atlanta. Chris is a fan, and he also started his own company where he would book different celebrities at these conventions.

"I'm coming out to meet with Disney about some stuff," he said. "I'd love to meet with you."

We got together at El Torito, a Mexican restaurant that's no longer there in Burbank, across from what used to be NBC Studios, which is now called something else, and he started easing me into the twenty-first century.

"I noticed you don't have a website," he said.

I also wasn't involved in Twitter, Facebook, none of that yet.

"I know what they are, but I don't know how to do it," I said.

I was trying to relight the fire under my work by seeking creativity and making myself relevant. In the past, what always seemed to work for me was action, moving forward, reembracing whatever it was that got me excited about doing all this performing and acting and singing in the first place.

I had to learn a voice lesson from my younger self. Here I was twice the age now, having to go through the learning process again: don't panic, Rob—remember what it was that got you out here. You're going to have to jump in with both feet, because that's the only thing that's ever worked for you.

I've got a USB microphone, I thought. *Let's plug it into my computer.*

"Let's call it *Talkin' Toons,*" I told Chris.

He said, "Great. I'll put it on iTunes for nothing, and we'll get you a Twitter account."

I did it, and damned if people didn't start listening. Fans would ask questions on social media: What's your favorite character? What's your favorite voice? What's your favorite episode? I'd answer them on the podcast. Soon I had more questions than I could provide answers for.

Sometimes my recordings were pretty bad technically, and I had to learn how to get better sound quality. I didn't even have the foggiest notion of how to monetize a podcast. I had literally just learned there were podcasts on iTunes.

Soon I worried that having just my voice on the show would get boring for the audience. So I called Maurice. We had talked about podcasts, and I said, "Hey, man, I'm learning that there's a giant *Pinky and the Brain* audience. I get so many questions on my podcast that are related to you and me and the show. Would you be my first guest on my podcast?"

He said, "Where do you want to do it?"

I said, "I'll come to your house."

I took my laptop and my microphone and sat at Maurice's kitchen table. It was decidedly low-tech. His dog barked. Somebody rang the doorbell, and Moe answered it. And we just kept recording. People loved it. We did some *Pinky and the Brain* stuff in the middle of it, and I had questions prepared that people had asked Maurice about the shows he'd done. It turned out to be, not surprisingly, the first hugely listened-to podcast episode I did.

The same chemical feeling returned, that feeling I would get from the first rock-and-roll band gigs in high school, or the first time I auditioned for a play and realized that I really killed it and that I would get a callback. Here I was at fifty-four years old, and all of a sudden I'm feeling the same butterflies about this thing called podcasting. People were digging what Maurice and I talked about. *Maybe I've got something here.*

Meantime, I started getting auditions again—first a trickle, then a stream. I had a renewed sense of purpose. I'd found a way to dig myself out of the hole without giving up. Well, not completely giving up. Maybe it was luck; maybe it was the usual ebb and flow of a career. But I think that the producers and casting directors could see that spark again.

Eight months later, I was back to working steadily. I did a show called *T.U.F.F. Puppy.* It was another longtime friend named Butch Hartman, a fellow Detroiter who was the creator of *Puppy* along with *The Fairly OddParents* and *Danny Phantom,* who got me the gig. God bless him.

Then my agent called and asked if I was aware that Nickelodeon's parent company, Viacom, had purchased the rights to everything Teenage Mutant Ninja Turtles. I said it sounded vaguely familiar, but I hadn't been paying that much attention to Hollywood deals during my downturn.

"They're casting a new version of the show," she said. "The producers were wondering if you would come in and read."

"Do they know who I was?" I asked.

My fear was that I'd get to the mic and only then they'd realize this was the guy who did Raphael in the original twenty-five years earlier. Everyone would be embarrassed for a second. They'd say some nice things, maybe throw me a bone in the form of a tiny little role, then we'd all go our separate ways.

"Yes," my agent said, "they know exactly who you are. They liked what you did with Raphael, and they thought you might be able to bring something interesting to Donatello this time."

I decided to audition using essentially my real voice, just like

Raphael. Raphael has a little harder edge, and Donatello is up higher, nerdier, but recognizable as me. I felt that if I was a good enough actor, the fact that one character sounded like another, even from the same franchise, wouldn't matter. I had a series of callbacks. And I got the job.

Sean Astin voiced my old character in the new cartoon. It was weird the first couple of sessions, seeing Raphael in the script and not responding when his lines came up. But Sean did an incredible job, and we soon fell into a rhythm.

When I booked *Turtles* in October of 2010, it started to occur to me that the fan base spanned two generations now. With the juice of Viacom and Nickelodeon behind the Turtles, I was going to be part of the biggest reboot for the franchise (at least at that time). My excitement had nothing to do with a paycheck. It had to do with finding new outlets for my creativity.

I had learned another voice lesson during this process of reimagining my career. When I'm able to fixate myself on long- and short-term goals, regardless of whether they come to fruition, oftentimes another goal will come up and take me off the main path. But that new goal is just as rewarding. Sometimes your goals change; sometimes you decide you don't want to reach the same goals again. But I found that after my real desperate period, action, any kind of forward action, was ultimately the secret.

What a gift, what a blessing, what a . . . whatever positive word you'd like to insert here. The main thing the new *Turtles* gig did was reassure me and cement the fact that I was back. I was back on my career path, with maybe even a new trajectory.

As lessons go, this one was painful enough but still came relatively cheap. I hadn't become that oldest of clichés, the Hollywood tragedy. I didn't miss any house payments or car payments. I fell behind on my taxes but had a plan to catch up.

I dug out of that nadir, and I'm very grateful to have found my way back, because I've embraced new technologies, new ways of being creative. It all conspired really well to be a good last act of my career.

It may not have been apparent at first, but the solution was as simple as getting up and saying, *I'm going to start making phone calls, I'm going to figure out podcasts, I'm going to make sure my agent knows I'm okay, whatever.* Going to a class, teaching a class, trying to create your own workshop, anything. I learned so much about just moving in a forward direction. After that action!

I continued to research live performing. At the time, Kevin Smith and Ralph Garman did a podcast called *Hollywood Babble-On* that streamed live from the Jon Lovitz Comedy Club. My friend Pat Brady, who was also a world-class voice-over agent, suggested that I do something at the club, too.

I had kicked around doing a one-man show until I saw James Arnold Taylor's show called "Talking to Myself" about his life as a voice actor. I'm smart enough to know what I'm not good at, and I knew I could never do a show that well. I loved singing more than anything, anyway. Countless times I had performed "Yakko's World" and other songs from *Animaniacs* a cappella at conventions and seen the reactions they always got. And one guy had written nearly all of those songs.

I had interviewed Randy on my regular podcast earlier. I called him and said they had an electric piano at the Lovitz. Maybe we could do an evening of *Animaniacs* songs?

The club welcomed us. Pat produced the show, and it was a blast. The audience loved it; the place was full. We started doing the show around town, at small parties and events for our friends. Then a fan of my podcast heard about our show and asked if we'd ever considered doing it with a big orchestra. He was friends with the conductor of the Colorado Symphony in Denver and offered to reach out. This had long been a dream of mine. I was inspired by the *Bugs Bunny on Broadway* shows at the Hollywood Bowl that combined animation with live orchestration.

One thing led to another, and in September of 2014 I was onstage with Randy, Tress, Jess, and an eighty-piece orchestra in front of twenty-five hundred people. To make it happen, Randy and I threw in some of our own money. Friends also invested. The Bernsteins helped us with the sheet music and all of the arrangements, updating the songs so that they could be played with up to eighty pieces.

The show was a big creative and financial success, and we were already dreaming of doing this around the world. We weren't a tribute band. We were the real deal, the folks who wrote and sang the music. I figured orchestras would be lining up to play with us. We put out the word to symphonies and cleared our calendars.

What we heard was crickets.

So we downscaled our plans and went back to doing clubs and small events, often for free. Randy and I wanted to use these gigs for experience. The Colorado concert had mostly been a string of songs. We wanted to build a show, something that was not only entertaining but informative, educational, and unique.

We worked up anecdotes between the songs to peel away the curtain and show the audience how the songs were inspired and written. We demonstrated what songs sounded like at first, then compared them to the finished product with orchestration and animation added. We performed songs that didn't make the cut on the show. We tailored the show for venues of varying sizes, from clubs to concert halls, from shows with just Randy, me, and a piano to full-blown performances with orchestras and other voice actors.

More gigs arrived, and the show was getting good and tight. I was energized. I loved voice acting, but it was liberating to find new and exciting ways to make it on my own, outside the recording studio, to have my mouth work for me for a change.

What I didn't take into account was the possibility that my mouth might have other ideas.

One of the first people I called was Randy.

I told him we'd have to put the show on the back burner.

CHAPTER NINE

Well, It's Cancer

I used to wonder what it would be like, really like, to find out I had a life-threatening disease. You see it on TV and in movies. The music swells, a look of horror crosses the face, tears fall, and the person crumples into a ball.

Some people say they don't react at all. Many talk about it as an out-of-body experience, as if they're watching it all happen to somebody else.

It was about 2:00 p.m. on a Thursday when my doctor called from Cedars-Sinai with the test results. He wanted to set a time for my wife and me to come to the office and discuss it. I said no. I live way the hell out on the western fringe of Los Angeles County. It would take an hour to drive to Beverly Hills. Plus I already had a good idea of what he was going to say.

I told him to just spit it out.

"Well, it's cancer," he said. "It looks like it's stage III. The full name is stage III squamous cell carcinoma with occult primary. And please do not get on the internet and look this up."

He explained that my kind of stage III cancer was different from other kinds of stage III cancer, like liver cancer or pancreatic cancer. It was specific to my condition and so would be my treatment. He repeated, over and over, that this was curable and that my prognosis was good.

He also assured me that the treatment—a combination of radiation and chemotherapy—would kick my ass.

The reality didn't take hold all at once. Nor did it sink in evenly over time. It was nonlinear. I'd be watching TV with my wife, and I'd look at her and I'd say, "Did you pick up milk today?" and then I'd think, *Oh, I've got cancer. In my throat.*

Then I would laugh. My wife would say, "Don't laugh, this is serious."

How could I not laugh? The irony of me getting throat cancer was inescapable. What's that old phrase—we make plans and God laughs? It was absurd. This was like being a place kicker and the doctor saying, "We have to remove your toe."

It was terrifying and silly and brought out my glib side. I would call up my doctor and be on hold, and when he finally answered, I'd say, "A guy can die of throat cancer while he's waiting for you."

I'd forget about it for a while. Then I would be driving along Ventura Boulevard and see a billboard about the number of cancer deaths from smoking, and I'd once again remember, "Wow, I've got cancer."

I'd drive by a hospital, and again I'd say, "That's me. I have cancer."

I would wake up, jump in the shower, and then all of a sudden think, *Wow, I've got cancer.* I'd be standing in a grocery line and see a magazine headline about "Val Kilmer's throat cancer nightmare." I would chuckle about our obsession with celebrity.

Then I would realize I'm having a Rob Paulsen throat cancer nightmare. Only it didn't feel like a dream. More like a strobe light of realizations.

I'd think of how people used to mention friends of ours who went to the doctor. I'd ask, "Oh, is he going to be okay?" And they'd say, "We're not sure, he's got cancer." I'd say, "That's awful."

Now I was going to be that guy they were talking about. I imagined the conversation:

"Did you hear about Rob Paulsen?" they'd ask.

"No, is he going to be okay?" I'd answer.

Wait, I am Rob Paulsen.

My out-of-body experiences were having out-of-body experiences.

Squamous cell carcinoma: I had heard that phrase because my father had skin cancer. The squamous cell variety is sort of an epithelial surface skin cancer.

I asked the doctor, "How did I get that in my throat?" I never smoked. I lived a healthy life.

"Well, we can discuss the possibilities," he said, "but essentially, you have the same thing that Michael Douglas had."

Wait, didn't he almost die? Or at least look like he did? Didn't he have a celebrity cancer nightmare that I saw on the cover of *People*? I vaguely recalled seeing footage on *Entertainment Tonight* of him sneaking in and out of a cancer clinic.

"So, it's not necessarily just on the surface of the skin," the doctor continued. "You can get a squamous cell carcinoma on the surface of an organ, if it's a mucus-covered area, like your throat, or you might get a squamous cell carcinoma on your lung, the surface of the lung itself, or your body cavity lining."

The cancer was metastatic, or spreading. The "occult" referred to the fact that the doctor didn't know yet exactly where the cancer cells were in my throat. That little camera, the exploration with his fingers, the fine-needle aspiration—none of it could pinpoint where the actual tumor was.

I underwent a PET scan, in which they shot me up with radioactive tracers to detect cancerous growth. The technician let me watch the results on a screen. The area of my throat around the lump lit up like a Christmas tree. That light said the cancer had spread. The best the doctor knew was that it was down there somewhere, deep.

"So we need to schedule you for a biopsy," he said. "I'm basically going to punch a bunch of holes in the base of your tongue and the back of your throat and take tissue samples, and then we can determine the margins of the cancer based on where the samples have been taken."

"Fire away," I said, glib as usual.

I was placed under general anesthesia. I thought I'd wake up and be in a sort of dreamy fuzzy world for a while, my own private Vicodin heaven.

Instead, they might as well have taken a rototiller to my throat. The pain was like nothing I'd experienced before. My son was next to me, holding my hand. I didn't want him to see me like this.

I kind of whispered, "Can you see if they can get me a shot or something?"

"Are you hurting?" he asked.

"My throat is hell."

Before the cancer, I had not felt one lick of serious pain, not like this. One of my most miserable things is mouth pain, for example, a sore throat or dental problems. I hate mouth pain because there's not much you can do about it—and I have to work with my mouth.

I remembered a few years back, when Michael Douglas went through his throat cancer, thinking that radiating your throat must be the worst thing possible. He was on *The Tonight Show* saying how brutal it was. I remembered that Roger Ebert had throat cancer, the same throat cancer I had. He wasn't as lucky as Michael Douglas.

So far in my treatment regimen, I'd only had a biopsy, and it was really tough. I had to send my son off to get me a shot of whatever the hell it was—Demerol, elephant tranquilizer, I didn't give a shit—just to get me home.

That's when it became real. I hadn't had one rad of radiation. I hadn't had one chemotherapy treatment. No vomiting, none of that stuff yet. All I'd had was a biopsy, and it was gnarly. If I hurt like that coming out of general anesthesia, I might not be able to handle what came next.

About two days later, the doctor called: "We've found the tumor. We got it. We know where it is. Now we're going to set you up with your radiation oncologist."

The radiation oncologist outlined my cancer game plan, a one-two assault on the cancer with radiation and chemotherapy. There would be seven weeks of radiation therapy, five days a week, Monday through Friday. It would take about a half hour once everything was set up. I would also be getting chemo treatments on Thursdays for eight weeks. I'd come in at 7:00 a.m. and be done by 11:30 a.m. or noon, a three- to four-hour drip.

"Your prognosis is excellent," he told me.

That was the good news. The bad news was they were going to strap me to a table every day and radiate my throat. I imagined Yakko and Pinky and Raphael and Donatello and Carl, poor sweet innocent Carl, all burned to a crisp.

After the biopsy from hell, it took me about a week before I could go back to work. The digging around took place in an area of my throat at the base of my tongue. But there was no nerve damage. It didn't damage my vocal cords. Once I could swallow water, I was good to go.

Up until this point, only a few people knew why I had taken sick leave. I spoke to my wife, and I said, "Okay. Here's the deal. There are certain people I have to let know."

Obviously, my siblings. I didn't want to worry them. But then, since cancer can run in families, I didn't want them to miss something that they should tell their own doctors about.

I told the producers of the two big shows I was working on, *VeggieTales* and *Teenage Mutant Ninja Turtles*. The producers were all understanding.

"You just get better," Doug TenNapel, the producer of *VeggieTales*, told me, "and I'll make it work at my end."

I told the producers that I knew and appreciated that they cared about me, but that I didn't know what was going to happen. I could finish recording the episodes that were in front of me, but I couldn't take on new episodes. I hoped that after the treatments I would sound good enough to do the job and finish up the seasons, but if they had to replace me, they shouldn't hesitate, and shouldn't feel bad. It's show business. It's not personal. I got that.

I also told Tress, Jess, Maurice, and Randy. That dinner with Sam Register from Warner Bros. was still weeks away. But we all had an inkling that *Animaniacs* might be returning.

These were tough phone calls. My fear was that the *Animaniacs* producers would want to bring back the entire original cast, or none of them. If they couldn't bring back the entire original crew, then maybe they'd get all new actors. I could have messed up everybody's gig. And these people are like my family.

But they made it easy on me. When I told them, one by one, about my cancer diagnosis, they were completely loving and sympathetic. They expressed no frustration or anger. They told me to worry about myself and my health and wait and see what happened with the show.

Meanwhile, my radiation started. The radiation oncologist was a younger guy, and we hit it off right away. He spoke in a thick Russian accent, like a James Bond villain, which gave everything he said a sinister edge. Over and over, he repeated how promising the long-term prognosis was, how small the chances were of the cancer returning once they fried it away, though his voice made even the best of news sound hopeless. My vocal cords would remain intact, he said. I would be able to speak again. Within two years I should be back on my feet.

But he warned me: the radiation treatment would get so bad that simply drinking a cup of water would feel like lava flowing down my throat. Eating would be pure torture. I'd lose a lot of weight. As for what musical notes I would be able to hit, what sounds I could affect, what accents and inflections and dialects I could conjure, nobody could answer that.

"My job is to save your life, not your career," he said in his Goldfinger voice. "I'm confident we can cure you. But first we're almost going to have to kill you."

He gave me the lowdown on the treatment and the machine that was going to zap me. I'm fascinated by that stuff and wanted to embrace this experience and learn. Confronting something and understanding it helps demystify it, especially if it frightens me.

He showed me a map of my neck, a three-dimensional image on the computer, and pointed out the tumor. They would have to be very, very specific with the beam of radiation. The machine would go around my head while I was lying still on a platform. To keep me from moving, they had to make a perforated plastic mask to hold my face and head.

They heated up this big piece of plastic with perforations in it. It was warm enough to be soft and pliable, but not hot enough to do any damage. I put my face in it. Much like a vacuum forming machine, it sucks the plastic right to your face. When it cools, it's just for you, and they put your name on it.

Every day I would come in and lie down. They would put the mask on me and bolt it to the table so that I couldn't move my head. I wouldn't even be able to open my eyes, because the mask was literally sucked to my eyelids. Nothing would move.

I would be able to breathe, of course, but I couldn't move my jaw. The technician would talk to me on the intercom, and I would communicate with hand signals. There was also a panic button.

The last thing the doctor explained was the concept of scatter. He would blast the tumor and also some of the area around it. His experience told him there would be random, teeny tiny cancer cells around the tumor. He wanted to get every one of them.

As the doctor talked, I flashed once again on Roger Ebert. He had the same cancer. That was what frightened me the most—going out in such a messy way. Talk about incredibly brave, Ebert and his wife. I wondered if I had the same courage.

I found a clinic for the radiation treatment ten minutes from my house. I wanted it close by, because I was determined to drive myself to as many of these as possible. I wanted to know that I could do it. I wanted to control this myself as much as I could. I wasn't going to ask anybody to drive me unless I was so sick I posed a danger to everybody else on the road.

Once my mask was made and my name was put on it, Dr. Goldfinger said, "We're ready."

On March 11, 2016, I turned sixty years old. The first treatments were scheduled to begin on March 21. I had ten days. Why not squeeze in some golf?

It was Patrick Warburton, of all people, who called me to play in his celebrity golf tournament. It took place at the JW Marriott Desert Springs Resort and Spa in Palm Desert, not far from Palm Springs, and it raised money for St. Jude Children's Research Hospital.

I asked my doctors if it was okay to play a few rounds, and they said this would be a good time. Once I began radiation treatments, I would have to do it every day, a serious commitment. If I missed a treatment, it would get tacked on to the end. I was told that the radiation and chemicals would do no favors for my golf swing. It was play now or wait months, possibly years.

I don't know Patrick well, but the Warburton Celebrity Golf Tournament is a big event and huge fund-raiser. A lot of rich people show up, writing checks for ten, twenty, thirty large to buy something autographed by Tiger Woods. It raked in $1.7 million that weekend. A lot of actors and musicians turned out, and there were several children and their families representing the wonderful work St. Jude does. The hospital doesn't charge anybody—all the legacy of Danny Thomas. They give children world-class treatment and never send them a bill.

Once I hit the course, everything was surreal. I couldn't concentrate. I didn't play well. I'm a good enough golfer to know how good I'm not. That's one of the best things about getting to be a pretty good amateur golfer—I really understand how impossible that game is, which is one of the reasons I love it. This weekend, my game didn't matter. I was there to have fun and raise money for the kids.

I was there with movie stars and rock stars and my little secret. I hadn't told Patrick or anybody at the tournament about my situation. My emotions were going crazy. I'd go back to my hotel room and lie awake and think, "Man, I'm hitting a golf ball and I'm laughing out there." And then I'd realize that we were working for St. Jude, and then I'd realize that we were working for kids with cancer, and then I'd realize, *Hey, I've got cancer.*

During the dinner/silent auction, there was a family onstage talking about one of their twin boys. The boy, who was about eleven, had felt crappy. The doctors ran tests, and before you know it, they find out he's got leukemia. That young man spent a year getting chemo every day, a year in the hospital. He was at the tournament with his brother and his mom and dad, all of whom, of course, had tears of gratitude in their eyes, thanking St. Jude, because there's no way they could have afforded it.

Listening to this family floored me. It contextualized my own upcoming treatment. After a few weeks, I was supposedly going to be cured. This kid went through it for a year.

I thought: *Okay, you really can do this, Rob. There are a lot of unknowns. But you are going to meet people who have been through the same thing, even worse, and survived.*

At the end of the weekend, I got to know a fellow who worked on behalf of St. Jude, a real sweet guy. We hit it off, and he said, "Man, I just love your work. I've been a big fan."

I thought about that boy and his family and said, "I've got to spill my guts about something."

He became the first person outside my immediate circle to know about the cancer. He put his arms around me and said, "I am so sorry, but I really feel like you're going to be okay."

"Me, too," I said. "I do really want to come visit St. Jude. I'm looking forward to having an opportunity to say, 'I get it. I'm one of you.'"

I've met many sick kids over the years. I've signed their posters and their jackets. I've tried to make them laugh. I've cried with their families after they died. I think I'm a fairly kind individual. I just love making people happy, and certainly making them feel good in a miserable circumstance with their children.

Not until now, however, did I begin to understand on a deeper level what they might be going through. I was always sympathetic. I thought now I could be empathetic.

I had been thinking to this point about cancer in terms of myself and my career, putting on a positive veneer for everybody around, trying to shield them from anything bad. The weekend had put me in a different frame of mind. I took my first baby steps toward letting go.

During a round of golf, I paused on the fairway and recorded a video of myself, a time capsule I could revisit—or, if things went south, somebody else could visit one day.

"Well, happy birthday to me," I told my camera phone. "I'm sixty years old today, and this is the first video I've made since I thought I might have cancer a couple weeks ago. I do. I'll be anxious to see how I respond to this video in a year. I'm currently at a fabulous golf tournament, thanks to Pat Warburton and his friends. This is kind of my last hurrah before all the fun begins with my cancer treatment. I consider myself an incredibly fortunate man for so many reasons."

I listed everybody I loved, starting with my wife, my son, Ash, and his wife. I listed Randy and Tress and Jess.

"Did I say Randy?" I asked the camera. My mind was starting to wander. "I love you guys, and I appreciate in advance what you're fixing to help me through. Let's light this candle. See you on the other side."

CHAPTER TEN

Zap Me

Before my first treatment, the doctors hooked me up with a social worker, a psychologist who encouraged me to express my feelings, any time, if I was freaking out. I'm a pretty cavalier guy, a pretty glib guy. Humor is a really important tool for me. The doctors encouraged this.

I found out later that all this accentuating the positive was the doctors' best effort to try to keep me on point. They gave me chapter and verse: look, we can help you, but we're telling you, Rob, that happy-go-lucky vibe that you are about, we don't want you to lose that. That is important.

They wanted to make sure I could try to look on the bright side when I was, say, puking. Or when I had taken so much pain medication I didn't know where I was. Or even when the nurse would come in and ask, without preamble, "Are you pooping?"

I was asked a lot about my poop, bowel movements apparently the window into the soul during treatment.

They would prefer that I joke with them if it gave them the information to understand what was going on and how I might need their help.

All of this I expected. What I didn't see coming was that this positivity encouragement can in some ways be a smoke screen. That's because they don't give you all the information up front, just enough to brace you for the bad but not pummel you with the possible worst.

If you knew the worst up front, you might just ditch the whole program and curl up in a corner.

From the start, I was told I would undergo hellish radiation and chemo that would destroy the tumor. It would be bad, very bad. They'd almost kill me. Got it, check. That biopsy got my attention. I understood.

I would then enter a recovery period that would more or less bring me back to normal, save for some weight loss and exhaustion. No guarantees on the cartoon voice, but I'd be vertical.

The first sense I got that there was more to the story was when I was referred to a speech pathologist. This was a little bit freaky at the beginning. I'd been speaking for money for the last thirty years, and now I may need somebody to help me talk?

I had been focused on the fact that the tumor hadn't spread to my vocal cords. I didn't count on having other long-term effects that might never go away.

This was the first time they told me about lockjaw.

When they started zapping my throat with radiation, it would leave adhesions, which, if not addressed, would become worse until I couldn't open my mouth. I had witnessed this before in another context, when my wife blew out a knee. She had a machine that exercised her knee for her even while she was sleeping, precisely because of the adhesions that would develop if her knee remained still. The machine had a pneumatic device that kept manipulating her knee at a certain level to maintain her range of motion.

If she didn't keep that up, they'd have to put her under with general anesthesia and do something the bone docs called "gross manipulation," bending her knee as far as it could go and popping these adhesions. It hurts like hell, so they knock you out.

Now imagine doing this in my mouth.

I needed to learn exercises that would break the adhesions in my jaw, a little at a time, as we went along. The therapist would tell me to grab on to my tongue and say, "A-E-I-O-U," then try to push my tongue as far as I could out of my mouth while keeping my mouth open. I would also try to touch my chest with my chin and move my head as far as I could to the left and the right and back. The therapist told me to do these exercises every day to help prevent my jaw from freezing up.

Apparently, they were concerned that if I wasn't stretching my jaw muscles as much as I needed to, the adhesions would do to my jaw what they had done to my wife's knee. The speech pathologist said it was not unlike an athletic endeavor, in which you have to warm up your muscles. I had to warm up my jaw the way a baseball pitcher warms up his arm. That scared me. They were very clear that this was important if I wanted to keep talking. They wanted to prepare my jaw, and they wanted me to do it every day.

You can bet your ass that I was vigilant.

One of the things that kept me focused and positive was my fascination with all the technology and its relationship with the body. I'm an armchair scientist, and I'm always kind of astonished at these machines that can keep us alive.

My mother had really awful kidney issues. She went to dialysis three times a week up in northern Michigan. A van would come by and pick her up, and she would go visit the good people at the dialysis center in Gaylord, Michigan.

I went to see my mother at dialysis probably half a dozen times. When you look at this giant machine and your sweet little four eleven, ninety-pound mother attached to it, you really get to see what a remarkable piece of meat a kidney is, what it does every day without us even thinking about it until we go to the bathroom.

I got to know her kidney doctor, who told me about my mom's condition. It turned out that her whole life, my mother only had one kidney that worked, and they didn't realize it until she started having these problems. My siblings and I discussed it, and we all offered to give her one of our kidneys.

"That's very sweet," the doctor said. "But your mother is eighty, and the surgery to remove the kidney and the surgery to implant the new kidney is both ethically and technically not a great idea."

The doctor then revealed that he'd already had this same conversation with my mother about a donation. I knew that she'd had a baby boy, born a year before I was born. In those days they had no amniocentesis, and they couldn't check things out like they can now. My brother had spina bifida. He lived two weeks.

The doctor said my mother didn't want a kidney from any of us. She didn't want to put another child at risk. It still chokes me up just thinking about it.

As I reflected on those treatments, I saw my own radiation machine in a new light. Sure, my head would be bolted to a table, but that beam of radiation would be able to do what no loved one ever could—tear up my cells to save my life.

My radiation treatments began the third week of March 2016 at 2:30 p.m. I was to go every day, Monday through Friday, for the next month. The doctors reminded me about the importance of sticking to the schedule. They told me I might be sore and exhausted and, when the chemotherapy began, vomiting, but that I should still make every effort to come. If I missed just one, they'd tack on an extra session at the end. It wasn't about the time, it was about the amount of radiation that I needed to kill the cells. When you get radiation, their empirical data suggests that you need to have this much radiation at this intensity specific to you.

I walked into the clinic, and the first thing they did was weigh me. They were very exacting about knowing what my weight was at every stage. I started at 178 pounds on a five-foot-ten frame. That was maybe ten pounds over my ideal weight, when I was at my peak playing hockey, but I was still in good shape. My heart rate at rest was like fifty-eight. I'm a weekend warrior. I've always been athletic.

The weight was important for a number of reasons. One was that every pound I shed could throw off the treatment plan. If I lost weight in my neck, the mask that held my head steady during radiation would not fit as well, and they'd have to recalibrate everything.

"We're ready for you, Rob," the technician said, and into the radiation room I went.

The tech asked me—as everybody seemed to—whether I needed to go to the bathroom. They didn't want me halfway into radiation and squirming because I had to pee. I said I was fine, then pressed my face into the mask and lay on the table faceup.

The mask was bolted to the table. My shoulders were locked, too—you can't move them for obvious reasons. You don't have to hold your breath, nothing like that. If you want to communicate, you have a buzzer in your hand, or you wave your hand or whatever and they'll stop the machine.

They left me alone, watching me on camera from another room. The person administering the treatment spoke over the PA system.

"You okay, Mr. Paulsen?"

I answered with a thumbs-up because I couldn't open my mouth.

The machine did its thing. In my case, they raised the platform, because the machine radiated me 360 degrees. The machine, supported by this big gantry, focused the beam. My eyes were closed and I couldn't see it, but I could hear it humming and buzzing.

You're like a big target. These are the margins, these are the areas, and as you get farther away from the target, the rads, the intensity of the radiation, is different and the color changes. So they know based on the color, hot or cool, where the most intense radiation is going. Every time they move you, I mean, a tiny little bit, they have to adjust the radiation.

I got to know the sound of the machine well within the first week. From the start to the finish, there were sounds that served as the audio road maps, letting me know that they were half-done, or there was ten minutes left. There was one specific sound, the best sound of all—a metallic buzzing. It meant the tech was repositioning the machine to the final location. Just two minutes left.

At first, the whole experience caused only mild discomfort. It completely fascinated me. I found that there was one special room off to the side of the machine room that was just used for cooling this device. The heat generated by the radiation is so profound they have to have another machine that cools that machine.

I began to wonder, What if I hear an "oops"? What if things start to shake and there's an earthquake while I'm on the table? Who's the knucklehead they bring in to fix this thing? I pictured a little guy in a cap and overalls who says, "Oh, we'll fix you right up, Mr. Paulsen. First, let me just go in and fix the cooling device. It's melting through to China."

My spirits stayed high. I got to know the guy pushing the buttons, a really smart guy who understands things I'll never comprehend. But I did learn enough about the technology to make my first physics joke.

I came in one day, and we were talking about how fascinated I was by the machinery. He was saying how one of the most famous doctors of physics in history is a guy named Max Planck, a peer of Einstein's, a German known for originating quantum theory.

"From now on," I told the tech, "I'd like to refer to the table as the Max Planck."

He smiled. "I am the only person you probably know in your life who would get that joke."

"That's why I did it, just for you," I said.

From then on, when I came in, he'd go, "Rob, do you want to lie down on the Max Planck?"

One day, somebody else at the clinic was in the room when he said it. The new guy said, "Oh my God. I get that," and suddenly I was the hit of the radiation lab. Not bad for an old turtle. They were saving my life, and I was making them laugh. I thought that was a pretty fair trade.

Fans, don't worry: I know that Max Planck joke wouldn't travel well, and I'd never dare try it onstage. Though when I told Randy before one of our gigs, shockingly, he got the joke. It seems he's into all that physics stuff, too. Who knew?

It was about two weeks into radiation when I first felt the effects—and at the worst possible time. It was when I bit into that steak at Morton's, when Tress, Jess, and I were meeting with Sam Register from Warner Bros. about a possible *Animaniacs* reboot. The radiation had attacked my taste buds; that fifty-seven-dollar porterhouse could have been medium-rare cardboard, making it impossible to ignore the cancer even as I was receiving the best news of my life.

This can't be happening, I told myself.

This was no regular cartoon gig. We're talking about a really big deal, *Animaniacs* and *Pinky and the Brain*, Steven Spielberg, Warner Bros., all of that. It was a life-changing show for me when it happened, and it's still the reason many people come to visit me at these conventions. The opportunity to get to do that show again with the same actors, with Mr. Spielberg, was just the kind of thing that every actor dreams of.

After the dinner, the other cast members supported me, of course, and said all the right things: that it was still early, we still hadn't gotten the official green light, there was no reason to shake things up yet. When we were in the parking lot after the dinner, all so excited, I said,

"I'm going to figure this out. One way or another, I will not let you guys down."

Warner Bros. essentially built my house, and that's not hyperbole. I owe these people a lot, and the very least I owed them was honesty and the respect to tell them the truth of my situation before they started the ball rolling. If there were any questions at all as to whether or not I'd be able to do this gig, I needed to be completely forthright before they spent a lot of money. I pride myself on being a fairly decent guy, and responsible. It was time to put that into action.

I called Sam. "I just want to be straight with you," I said. "About a month ago, I was diagnosed with stage III throat cancer."

I briefed him on the state of my treatment and the probable recovery schedule. I told him it hadn't spread to my vocal cords, but the doctors couldn't make any promises about how my voice would endure treatments.

There was a silence.

"Rob, I'm so sorry," he said.

"Sammy, thank you, and I believe you," I said. I thanked him for the dinner, for making us feel like movie stars.

"You are," he said. "You guys are a big deal."

"Yeah, but we're rank-and-file actors," I said. "This sort of shit just doesn't happen all the time, so thank you."

He kind of laughed, and said, "Great timing, huh?"

All I could say was "Yeah."

"Well, nothing's going to happen right away," he said. He didn't ask me questions I couldn't answer. He didn't say anything that indicated to me that he was the least bit concerned, or upset, or that he thought it might be a problem. Nothing. He was not only professional but utterly supportive. He really did take a lot of pressure off me by being so generous with his concern.

He told me the general thought was the show might happen within six months to a year. "Let's just see how it shapes up," he said. "Your first job is to be okay, and then we'll see what happens."

And that's where he left it. I went back to my treatment. He checked in every now and then. We would just wait and see.

As my radiation treatments progressed and my chemotherapy sessions began, a dry mouth now conspired with my inability to taste to make my mouth a wasteland. A nagging fatigue had begun to worsen to bouts of exhaustion. In a word, I felt crappy. I knew I had to tell more people about my cancer. The most difficult calls I had to make were to three of my closest friends, the other original Ninja Turtles: Cam Clarke, Barry Gordon, and Townsend Coleman.

We had been there at the beginning, made hundreds of hours of cartoons together. We had visited sick kids in hospitals. We'd gone through the disappointment of being shut out of the movies. Although I was the only one brought back for the new incarnation of *Turtles*, we continued to do public appearances together, the fan base always excited to meet the original cast.

We'd do panel discussions and pose for photos. We had recently been in Calgary, us four plus Renae Jacobs, who was the original April O'Neil, and Peter Renaday, who was the original Master Splinter. Each of us would have lines, really long ones, of parents and their children dressed up as Ninja Turtles.

At the time of my diagnosis, we had convention appearances booked through the end of 2016. The next one was set for Indianapolis. I felt physically up to the show, but I knew I couldn't miss three or four days of radiation or I'd have to tack on more at the end, when my body would be ravaged by the upcoming chemotherapy.

"Look, I just want to let you guys know," I told them. I explained that I'd been diagnosed with throat cancer and had to back out of at least four appearances.

I don't ever, ever want to hurt somebody's ability to make a living. Work like ours is too hard to get under the best of circumstances. I worried that if the conventions didn't get all four Turtles as promised, they'd cancel the whole gig for everybody. To a Turtle, the guys responded with warmth and understanding. "I love you," they said, and I could tell they meant it. Every one of them was perfect. Just perfect. They could not have handled it better.

Then I invented a cover story.

Through my representatives, I told the conventions that I had strained my voice from too many recording sessions and didn't want to end up with a career-ending node on my cords. In other words, I lied. To be brutally frank, I didn't have any reluctance doing it. I didn't want to make a bad situation worse.

News like mine has a way of spinning out of control with fans, many of whom are very devoted to their favorite cartoons. It's not a large leap from "Oh my God, Rob Paulsen has been diagnosed with cancer" to "Rob Paulsen is dying." Or dead.

I didn't want to give anybody reason to worry. Many of my fans are children. And this was all difficult enough for me to process.

I knew, as my body was going to weaken from the treatments, that I'd be too exhausted to knock down each and every incorrect tweet or Facebook post. I had to focus on my health while doing everything possible to save my career. So I was willing to tell a lie.

The other practical reason for the fib was that I didn't want to give anyone in Hollywood a reason not to hire me. Even if their reasoning might have been in deference to me.

I have a wonderful friend, a casting executive, who went through brain cancer and came back to work. I knew he would be one of those guys who would understand, and I've since had a couple of really nice chats with him about what it's like to take a punch in your head and in your throat. But not everybody was like him. Not everybody would understand. They might have the best of all intentions, thinking they were helping me by leaving me alone, but I didn't need them worrying about my health when I had recovered and was ready to get back to work.

I promised myself I'd set the record straight as soon as I could. The message was going to be "I told a lie, here's why. If you can forgive me, great. If you can't, great, but I have my reasons."

Aside from the producers, I kept pretty quiet. It meant biting my tongue when I would hear people say, "Yeah, I'm sorry I'm late. My mother is having chemotherapy. She's got breast cancer." It was very difficult for me not to chime in and say, "Oh man, I've got cancer, too." Instead, I'd say, "Oh my gosh. Well, please know that you're in my thoughts, buddy. I'm so sorry."

I was determined to keep working as long as possible during radiation. I thought I was being a trooper, proving something to myself, trying to exert some modicum of control.

I wanted to tell cancer, *fuck you*. I started my once-a-week chemotherapy sessions. And cancer said *fuck you* right back.

CHAPTER ELEVEN

Pinky and the Brain
Take Over the Cancer Ward

Everybody was assigned a nurse to administer the chemo. The sweet lady who was to help me with mine was laughing at my voices and dumb jokes. "Gosh, Rob. Good for you," she said. "You're going to be fine." This was during a prep day, shortly before my first actual treatment.

Then she closed the curtains around the two of us. She sat down on a swivel chair and pulled up to me.

"Okay, hotshot," she said. "We've got to have a serious talk."

I did a double take.

"What you're doing and the way you're behaving is all great, and keep it up because"—then she put her hand on my leg—"honey, you're going to need it. You're going to get through this, no doubt, with flying colors. The way you relate to the other people and the staff, keep it up.

"But also, when you don't feel like it, don't do it, because there's going to come a time when you're going to come in here and you're not going to want to make anybody else happy. Remember, Rob, this is about you. You're dealing with something that will kill you if you don't treat it."

"No, I understand that."

"Good," she said. "Now, I also need to talk to you about some stuff that's really personal, and some people handle it well and some people don't, but I've got to tell you."

I felt on safer ground now. Self-consciousness has never been an issue with me. If three decades in show business has taught me anything, it's that a reckless disregard for anything approaching dignity can take you far as a cartoon voice actor.

"We're doing the first chemo the typical way," she said. "We tie you off, we find a vein, and off we go. As we progress with the other chemo sessions, they're about three- or four-hour treatments once a week for eight weeks. I need to tell you that once you have your chemo treatment, for about twenty-four hours afterward, everything that comes out of your body, and I mean everything, is toxic."

I said, "What?"

"I'm going to give it to you straight. When you get sick and throw up, if you can't make it to the toilet and you throw up on the floor, make sure that your dogs don't get near it, and make sure that you clean it up and then wipe everything up with Clorox, and then dispose of whatever you used to clean it up in a separate bag, and take it out and put it in the garbage by itself."

"Are you kidding me?"

"No," she said. "By the same token, if you have your own toilet, do not let your wife or your son use it, unless you clean the toilet yourself after you use it every time."

"Are you kidding me again?"

"No, because we don't want any possibility. Your urine is toxic."

Thirty years in the cartoon business, and I'm finally a character out of Marvel comics. And my superpower is peeing chemicals. I'm radioactive. I'm like the Toxic Avenger. The crazy Ninja Turtle from Three Mile Island. Talk about happy ooze.

"That's not to harsh your mellow," the nurse said. "Keep it up. But we just need to tell you, and that's also why we really think you should get the port in your arm. We don't want to spill it on your skin."

She suggested I install a spigot in my body. That way they wouldn't have to always look for a vein to pump in the chemo. By the fourth or fifth time, it would be a mess. I readily agreed.

I went in for an outpatient procedure. They made an incision into the deep vein in my arm and then inserted a tube that fed up to my heart so they could pump the chemo directly into my ticker. It would avoid spillage on my vein or the surface of my skin.

It was a little uncomfortable getting it, but I was mesmerized by the treatment. They did it with a fluoroscope—the doctor watched in real time as he was feeding the tube into my heart. I said, "I want to watch you do this."

They brought over the fluoroscope, and they were able to position it over my chest while I watched it with the surgeon who did this implant. He said, "Here it comes," and there was this little tube right on the screen, and it stopped at my heart, which I could see pounding. It was amazing.

They sewed me up and left a little rubber thing under my skin. When they inserted the treatment or whatever, it was just like getting a shot. It hurt for a nanosecond, but that was it. It was the best decision I made.

On my first day of chemo, I tried to keep my attitude positive.

"All right," I said, "fire me up. Let's kill this stuff."

As cavalier as I was and as positive as I am, when I was sitting there, I couldn't help thinking about the other patients, many of whom were not going to live to finish their chemo. Yet they still had courage and grace and a sense of humor.

"Hey, Morty?" one man said to another. "How are you doing?"

"Ah, I've only thrown up twice."

I would see this lady, who was really getting hammered with chemo, and yet she was just so effusive and outgoing. "I've been here a couple of times," she said. "I know what I'm talking about. How you doing, honey?"

I later told another patient, "That woman is so courageous."

"This is all palliative care," the other patient said. "She's on her way out."

She's on her way out, but not without making sure a couple people laughed. Whenever I would feel afraid or nervous or whatever, humor was my default mechanism, too. Humor was where I could go to relax, my version of a mantra. Humor made me feel more comfortable, because I'd been doing that for sixty years. It was my own medicine. It was my balm—a balm for my soul.

And if anybody asked, sure, I told them what I did. Pinky and Yakko and Raphael came to the chemo clinic. People would come up and say, "Could you say, 'Turtle power' to my kid?" They'd say, "Hey,

I think we're not supposed to do this, but my girlfriend is crazy about *Pinky and the Brain*. Would you record her a message?"

Of course I would. It was really cool that we were all giving each other things that were important. I think it helped me more than the other patients, bringing out my favorite characters. That was my spoonful of sugar. It did help the medicine go down, whether it was in my arm or in my mouth, and it turns out it helped other people, too.

I was already in the chair on one of my Thursday chemo treatments when I got a text from Maurice.

"Hey, buddy. I'm in the neighborhood. You want a visitor?"

I knew damn well that it wasn't like he just happened to be driving down Wilshire and ended up outside the clinic. It was so good to hear from him.

"Oh my God, that would be great," I said.

Seeing Maurice would be a kind of normal occurrence, or a sense of normalcy, in a very odd circumstance—me in my chemo chair, hooked up to a tube. I was trying to take it all in stride, and I think I was doing a pretty good job of it. But having a dear friend there, who knew me really well, gave me a sense of comfort and joy.

Plus, I knew that when he got there, we'd both want to play.

Maurice took a seat next to me while the chemicals poured into my body. We got to joking. And pretty soon, one thing led to another, and somebody said, "Hey, you know who these two guys are?"

Pinky and The Brain were in the house.

It happens all the time when Moe and I are together. If we're walking through an airport together, it happens at TSA. You get these people who are just doing their job, and it can be very boring. Inevitably, Maurice knows how to light the candle.

"Greetings, my friend," he'll say in his Orson Welles–Brain voice. The person will look up and not quite get what's happening. I'll kind of roll my eyes, and I'll say, "I'm so sorry about my friend. Do you watch cartoons?"

"Yeah, sure, I guess."

"You ever watch *Pinky and the Brain*?" I'll ask.

"Oh, yeah, sure."

Moe will say, "That's Pinky," and I'll give them a squeaky Cockney, "How ya doing, Officer Johnson?"

And they immediately light up. I don't care if it's Canadian customs. I don't care if it's US customs. I don't care if it's TSA at Cleveland, LAX, Charlotte, Chicago. They all love it. It happened the other day, a couple of weeks ago at the time of this writing, when Moe and I were in the Admirals Club at O'Hare coming back from a show. We walked in. Maurice is a member of their Admirals Club.

We were probably talking a little too loudly and giddily, and I finally told a woman sitting there, "You'll have to excuse him. He's a little bit dim."

And then, of course, I started playing around. She kind of laughed, being polite.

"I'm so sorry," I said, "we're tired. We just got done working at this Comic-Con."

"Oh, really. What do you do?"

Cue: playtime. Pinky and The Brain are in the Admirals Club.

"Are you kidding me?" the lady said. "Can I get a picture with you and Mr. LaMarche? Oh my God!"

Every time, so help me God, we can't help it. We're actors. It's in my blood, more powerful than that cancer-killing juice. And so, I knew that was going to happen at the hospital. I prefer to think it's the joy I derive from doing it. It's probably my ego. Still, it's so much fun.

I was already feeling pretty good anyway. That chemo cocktail is full of steroids. I was amped.

The truth is, Moe and I not only love each other, but we kind of need each other. I couldn't do *Pinky and the Brain* with anyone else, and I truly believe Moe couldn't do it with anyone else. If the worst had happened and I'd checked out, I think that would've been it for Moe, too. He wouldn't have done The Brain anymore.

Moe and I have spent as much time making people laugh for no money as we've spent getting paid for it. Probably more. It happens with fifteen-year-olds, and it happens with seventy-year-olds.

So here we are at the chemotherapy room, and I'm singing, and Moe is going to take over the world, and it's wonderful. It was more therapy for me than the other people, the most incredibly wonderful experience that no one else can create, no one but Maurice and me.

By the fifth week, the side effects from the radiation intensified. I was getting more tired. My mouth was drier. I was still very positive, but I found myself experiencing more intense emotions at the most unexpected times.

I was driving home one day from a chemo treatment and there was an accident on the freeway, so I took a side route down Sherman Way. I was in a new fancy, snazzy car, another one of my respites. If I had to go to chemo, I'd go in a bitchin' ride.

I turned up the music, trying to take my mind off my chemo pain. Then I saw this woman who looked to be, I don't know, fiftyish. She was crossing in front of me at the light, dragging her big bag of recyclables behind her. I don't know if she was homeless, but she certainly was a woman with some problems.

This was when I was just starting to feel crappy from the radiation. I snapped to attention: she didn't make eye contact with me and never will.

And I had this inner conversation with myself: What if she were in my position? Where is she going to go to feel as bad as I do? Where is she going to go when she can't drink anything? Where is she going to go when she throws up all over everything and her vomit is toxic?

I'm driving home in a BMW M6 to my beautiful home, to a wife and a son who are pulling out all the stops to make sure I'm comfortable in a king-size bed, and all my world-class doctors are going to give me whatever I need to get through it.

When I get home tonight and start to feel like shit, I can drop a couple of Vicodin and turn on Pink Floyd. I took a moment to really understand how incredibly fortunate I was on so many levels, even when I was facing the most difficult challenge of my life.

And not just *my* life.

Parrish was very frightened, and obviously wanted to make sure she got everything right. I mean, she got it more than right. But it was hard on her. In fact, later, when I was really struggling to stay conscious from all the medication, she was struggling much more than I was. I spent that month pretty much in a state of Vicodin bliss. She and my son didn't have that luxury.

The one advantage we had, if you want to call it that, was that my wife had endured her own cancer ordeal. The lumpectomy and radiation cured her breast cancer, but as anyone who has undergone radiation knows, she was never 100 percent the same again. She knew what I was in for, keeping on me with the pain medication and the nutritional supplements. She knew when to worry, and she knew when to panic, like the day I stood up too quickly and the next thing I knew I was waking up on the floor with a ding in my forehead, and with Parrish shaking me and saying my name.

As I came to, I insisted I would be fine in a minute, but she overruled me and called the paramedics. She wanted to make sure I hadn't suffered a stroke. An ambulance took me to the hospital, where the doctors said I'd probably had a sudden drop in blood pressure. But having my wife act quickly put my mind at ease. She was much better in a crisis than I was.

The effects of the chemotherapy were more fleeting than the radiation. For about two days after each chemo session, I actually felt pretty good. I got this chemo buzz. "Wow, I feel great with the steroids."

Then on Saturday morning after my chemo, I crashed. I had this awful taste of metal in my mouth from the platinum-based chemicals. I would want to eat, but I would take a bite or two, and I just couldn't. It didn't taste good. Whatever I ate tasted like the chemo. The first couple of times I was still able to eat something and keep it down. They gave me all kinds of antivomiting stuff. Sometimes it worked, sometimes it didn't, but at least I had something in my stomach—because I had something to throw up. I threw up a lot. Two days of throwing up.

But by the third treatment, I simply couldn't eat. Then came the dry heaves. The heaves would not stop. It was exhausting. They wrapped my whole body up. I couldn't control them. The heaves flexed every muscle, and I ached everywhere.

The sickness from the chemo would go away by Monday, and I would still try to drag myself to work. But the side effects from the radiation got worse. My mouth was becoming a war zone. The mucosa lining my throat was obliterated from the radiation.

A dry mouth led to a risk of infection. They gave me something they called Magic Mouthwash. It's a combination of different antibiotics. The Magic Mouthwash is really great because it helps mitigate the pain. You get all sorts of sores in your mouth from the radiation. If you know what a bad canker sore feels like, it's like that—and a whole lot worse. Imagine two months straight of strep throat. Every glass of water felt like Tabasco sauce searing open wounds.

My jaw began to ache. I had to go see an oncological dentist because of the way the bones in my jaw were compromised by the radiation. I couldn't take Vicodin during the day because of the side effects. But as long as I had some mouthwash or saltwater stuff, I could at least get to the place where I was able to do my work.

Part of my reason for continuing to work was that this was my way of saying, "I can do this." I didn't want to give in. Nobody really had a problem with the way I was sounding. I told myself: "Dude, you're not living under an overpass. You can do this." Other people had it worse and kept going.

I thought again of my little buddy Chad, who had become one of the biggest inspirations to me.

After meeting him, I had gotten involved with the Muscular Dystrophy Association of southern Alberta because they worked with his family, and his family essentially took me on as an adopted son. They could not have been nicer, and we exchanged addresses and phone numbers. I would call Chad and his sisters, Mandi and Jennifer, one of whom also had muscular dystrophy. And I kept in touch with all of them: Christmas cards, phone calls, etc.

As a result, I got a call a couple months after I met Chad from one of the folks who headed up the Muscular Dystrophy Association there in Calgary. He said, "Chad and his sister Mandi are our poster children this fall. Would you come up and host the Calgary feed of the telethon?" They had a local newswoman as a cohost.

I knew I could think on my feet in a live broadcast. So I did it. For four years in a row. I went up and hosted the Calgary feed of the telethon, appearing whenever they would break away from the telethon in Las Vegas hosted by Jerry Lewis. I'd join Chad on camera, and we'd sing the *Ninja Turtles* theme song. It was just great. His family would come on and say far too many nice things about me. And I'd say, "I'm the one that should be grateful." And I was.

Every time I was done with the telethon, I was an absolute mess, exhausted but feeling like I'd at least done something to make a difference. I would get ready to jump in the car to go back to the airport, and I'd look back at Chad's family. I'd wave goodbye, and they would be smiling and telling me how much they love me.

And I knew: they were going home with two kids in wheelchairs. They did it every damn day and never thought twice—at least outwardly—about doing it. But they're only human. There had to be points every so often where they thought, I cannot. I cannot clean up one more mess. I cannot bang the hell out of my little boy's back one more time to loosen up the phlegm, to keep him from pneumonia. I cannot hear my son say one more time, "Mommy, it's too hard, it's too hard." All the while knowing their kid was only going to live to twenty, if he was lucky.

They were tireless. They were heroes. Chad and his family inspired me throughout my ordeal.

But there came a point when I, too, was only human. I was still working on *Ninja Turtles*, *VeggieTales*, and *Doc McStuffins* for Disney. I tried to not book anything on the days when I had chemo and radiation on the same day, but otherwise, I would try to be done with work every day by 3:00 p.m. so I could make it back to my radiation treatment.

By weeks five and six, I had issues with my dry mouth and with taste. I was chewing all sorts of gum that would give me more saliva. I was losing weight, not precipitously but steadily—about six or seven pounds so far. It was from not eating, not really caring about eating.

Finally, my physical circumstance trumped my desire to work. It was time for me to concentrate on what was going on now.

In May of 2016, I bade farewell to all the little characters who had meant so much to me, who had taken me so far, who had amused me, enlightened me, who had fed my family and built my house and made me the person I was.

I needed the break, and I would have been useless. As bad as I thought it was now, it was only going to get worse.

CHAPTER TWELVE

High Times

One of the many cruel jokes of cancer treatment is that just as the treatments make it nearly impossible to keep food down, you start burning more calories.

A normal metabolism would go through about six hundred calories a day just surviving, processing food, walking to and from the car, keeping the heart beating. But with the assault from the radiation, my metabolism was now at about fifteen hundred calories a day, just existing.

So even though I couldn't taste anything, couldn't swallow, couldn't hold down food, and barfed up what little got down my throat, I needed three thousand calories to keep my weight up.

When was the last time I ate three thousand calories a day? That's what you eat at Thanksgiving, and that's if you have, like, three helpings. That's four meals a day at the Cheesecake Factory. And then the next day you're absolutely stuffed.

The doctors set me up with a nutritionist who gave me recipes for shakes, most of which my wife made. The daily drumbeat from the nutritionist was, "You are going to lose twenty-five to thirty pounds, minimum. And if you don't keep up your nutrition, you're going to have a problem. You're not going to die, but you could have other issues."

I tried, Lord, I tried, but I couldn't eat. I hadn't realized the inextricable link between my ability to taste food and my ability to desire food. I thought that my body would crave nutrition, that I would get hunger pangs and wouldn't give a shit that I couldn't taste it. It didn't work that way for me. If I couldn't taste anything, I didn't care.

My wife would push me: "Well, I don't give a shit if you don't care, you have to drink it."

And I would, and then I would gag, and goodbye, shake.

The doctors kept pushing for calories, any calories. They didn't care if it was nutritionally lacking. If it meant drinking fourteen Slurpees from 7-Eleven or eighteen Frappuccinos from Starbucks, do it. Even my nutritionist admitted that while she preferred I drink coconut milk with olive oil and avocado, I should find those calories anywhere I could.

When it came to the point where the rubber met the road, the doctors took me aside and admitted as much. All that shit they tell men my age not to eat? Eat as much of it as you want. If I could find a way to get a piece of cheesecake down, do it.

Thank God for Ensure and Boost. To old folks and to infirm folks who are compromised, sometimes they're the only things that give you enough energy to go to the bathroom. I first considered Ensure absolute shit, empty calories. But later I was able to get those Ensures down because they were little eight-ounce bottles and they were thick and creamy. I couldn't taste it anyway, so I could get it down before I gagged. I could suck back one or two and then hold my breath and try to calm down, keep it down. That was the best I could do.

In my endless quest for calories, I would have an extra-large chocolate malt from Baskin-Robbins, which was about a thousand calories. Or a giant something from Jamba Juice with peanut butter and chocolate and anything else they could throw into the blender.

But there was no way I could drink three of those in one twenty-four-hour period. I just couldn't do it. At the best, I was maybe five hundred calories to the good each day. The weight loss began to become precipitous.

Early in my treatment, one of my doctors warned me about the weight loss and said one option was to install a feeding tube. The doctor had recommended against it, suggesting a more conservative approach of trying to eat on my own. But as I started wasting away, I wanted to hook one of those things up now. Plug me in and mainline those calories. Unfortunately, it was too late for the procedure.

I was down fifty pounds. And that was too much. The doctors were quite concerned, not that I was going to die, but that I'd have real trouble with too much muscle loss. The fat is one thing, but I was starting to lose muscle, and that's when it really starts to mess with your head.

I would stand in the mirror and look at the flaky skin on my arms. I tried to be cavalier about it. I'd joke I hadn't worn skinny jeans like this since seventh grade. But when I saw those dark circles under my eyes, my collarbones sticking out, I just broke down.

People would notice. It would happen at the drugstore and the grocery store, places where, before, when they found out who I was, I'd break out a cartoon voice and everybody would be happy. Now they would pat me on the shoulder and ask, "Are you a patient?"

"I am," I'd say.

And they'd say, "Oh, I went through it," or "My wife went through it."

I appreciated it, but this was a jarring turnaround. I was used to being the caring, benevolent semicelebrity who would parachute into a charity event or children's hospital and express genuine concern for the kid in the wheelchair. I was the one who would so graciously sign a jacket or volunteer for a fund-raiser, then fly home to my sports cars and hit TV shows.

Now I was the one who people were coming up to and saying, "God bless you, my friend."

After a while, I couldn't even hold down the shakes or the smoothies or the Ensures. Finally, I couldn't keep water down. One sip would send me to the bathroom heaving. An ice cube prompted waves of nausea.

First weight loss, now dehydration. The doctors said I would either have to go to the emergency room every day to get an IV drip to stay hydrated, or take care of it myself at home.

I opted for home care. I already had the little port they used for the chemotherapy. A nurse could come to the house and just plug in some saline. Hydration problem solved.

I had sunk so low that this news made me feel like I'd found $1,000 stuffed in a jacket pocket. It would all be paid for thanks to my health insurance, available due to my membership in the Screen Actors Guild.

Thank you, for the millionth time, Frings.

A nurse came over every day, early, at 6:30 a.m. I would get out of bed and make my way out to the TV room so my wife could sleep, turn on the tube or pop in a DVD, and get juiced up. The whole process seemed simple enough, so I asked the nurse if I could do it myself.

"If you don't mind?" he said.

"Drop me off a case of this stuff," I said.

He showed me how to do it. I had to purge the little thing with a squirt of something, put the IV drip in, and immediately I would taste lemons. The stuff I squirted into my arm made me taste lemons. It was so bizarre. The body is such a phenomenal, complicated machine.

I took my fluids while sitting in a chair in the TV room and watching DVDs.

One of my good friends is Butch Hartman, a fixture of Nickelodeon for twenty years and a fellow Detroiter. He created *The Fairly OddParents*. He created *Danny Phantom*. I met Butch at Hanna-Barbera, when he and Seth MacFarlane both had deals there. They wrote for a show called *Johnny Bravo*.

I was working with Butch on a show he created called *T.U.F.F. Puppy* when I told him about my cancer diagnosis. We were nearing the end of recording for the series, but I was still part of the show, and I wanted to let him know what was going on. He'd hired me, probably when he could've made a better choice. But Butch was always, always in my corner.

I told Butch I was going to be fine, but it was going to be tough for a few months. The next day, at my front door, I got the complete set of *I Love Lucy* and *The Office* on DVD. He knew that I was going to be in a position where I needed to be cheered up. I was touched. I was grateful. And I ended up watching every season with that saline drip.

One of the most beautiful things about my two rides in the Turtle van, so to speak, has been watching how the fans respond to the characters—their teamwork, this brotherhood, the way the Turtles have all got each other's back, how they fight and they pull pranks on each other like kids but ultimately they are totally there for each other.

When Donatello's got his shell up against the wall, he knows that at the last minute his Turtle brothers are going to come in and beat up the bad guys and get him to safety. But it turns out, it's not just on the show. A couple of times a week, I'd get texts from Sean Astin: "Are you okay, buddy?" "How you doing, brother?" "Can I come over?"

I worked with his father, John, many times before I got to know Sean, and they're lovely people. His mother was Patty Duke, the star of a popular sitcom who became an outspoken advocate for people with mental illness at a time when few people spoke publicly about it, after she was diagnosed with bipolar disorder. I found her honesty refreshing and heroic. After she passed away in 2016, Sean picked up the cause for her.

As much respect as I had for Sean, I couldn't help but rib him now and then. We sat next to each other in the recording studio for 120 episodes of the *Turtles* reboot, and if he ever struggled with a line as Raphael, I'd tell the director, "If Sean can't handle it, I'm happy to give it a shot."

Thankfully, he didn't hold it against me. When my shell was against the wall, he was there.

Well hydrated and caught up on my shows, I turned back to the problem of calories. The doctors continued to give me the green light for bad eating. Even booze. "That is, if you feel you can get a shot of vodka down," one doctor said, then reminded me of what it may feel like to splash alcohol on raw, ravaged skin.

No, thanks.

Desperate times called for funky measures. To a person, every one of my doctors was fine with me turning to marijuana to increase hunger and tamp down the nausea. There's certainly enough empirical evidence to suggest that medical marijuana has incredible benefits, on so many levels, for so many people struggling. Since this was before California had approved recreational pot, I had to get a doctor's card for medical marijuana, which was as easy to get in California as avocado on toast.

My wife drove me to a doctor in Santa Monica who specializes in green treatment. The doctor explained the different kinds of pot and their active ingredients, the THC versus CBD. He suggested something heavy with CBD, or cannabidiol, which helps calm you down, helps you with your appetite, but doesn't have the mind-blowing effects of pot. THC, or tetrahydrocannabinol, is the one that helps you get stoned. He recommended a ratio of one part THC to five parts CBD. So you have to take a lot of it to get high, but very little of it to help you with your appetite. Just a few little drops on the tongue.

Full disclosure: I had smoked pot a few times when I was a kid. Of course, it was illegal in those days, and you'd have to find a guy who knew a guy who'd score you some weed. I never got into it. It stank. I didn't like the feeling. It just made me go to sleep.

Now they were selling the stuff out of a storefront dispensary. The pot was beautifully marketed and regulated. Along with the usual buds, they had it inside strawberries and blueberries and gummy bears (I'll never look at that cartoon gig the same way again). It was very clearly listed as to what the percentages of CBD and THC were in each product.

In walked in, this old Ninja Turtle. Cowabunga, dude! I can buy dope!

I kept looking at my wife, going, "How crazy is this?" My "budista" had all these nose rings and earrings and tattoos and a Pink Floyd shirt. He said, "Hi, my name is Sunshine. I'll be your dispensary professional for today. Do you wanna buy a Blue Kush? Or do you want to buy Tangerine Dream? Or do you want to buy Jerry Garcia?"

"No, no, no," I said, "I don't want to get stoned."

Well, maybe a little stoned. I don't know. This was new to me. I explained that I was a cancer patient and told him the name of my doctor, and the budista lit up, metaphorically speaking, and pointed me to the right stuff.

"Why don't you get some of these chocolate-covered blueberries," my wife suggested, "because it looks like you only need to eat one?"

If they were chocolate covered, maybe they'd just melt in my mouth and I wouldn't have to worry about trying to swallow them. I flashed my card, shelled out some cash, and did what would have gotten me arrested back in high school.

When I got home, I popped two pot berries in my mouth. And, oh my God, all of a sudden I was Wavy Gravy at Woodstock. I mean, I was gassed.

Then I went right to sleep. Just like high school.

Did it make me hungry? Not that much at first. I still had trouble getting food down. I still had issues with my appetite. Mostly it helped with the discomfort and gave me a respite from the pain. It also made *Real Housewives* a *lot* more interesting.

I also tried the CBD oil that I applied with a dropper on my tongue. Since it didn't have the psychoactive ingredients, it didn't make me stoned, but it did help me sleep. And since I was struggling to keep down food, the little drop of oil worked better.

But not even the pot could address the worst of the side effects, which were starting to get ridiculous. One evening I started hiccuping. Normally if you hiccup and can't stop, you drink water and it subsides. This didn't work for me. I couldn't keep the water down. And the hiccuping continued. It went on for *two* hours. It was really hurting. People break ribs from this.

I called one of my doctors, and in between hiccups told him my problem. He chuckled and said, "I'm so sorry."

"Is this okay?" I hiccuped.

"It's not okay because it hurts," he said, "but it's not dangerous. We can fix it."

He explained that sometimes the vagus nerve, or whatever nerve it is that causes that involuntary response, gets tickled or gets a little bit tweaked by the radiation. It gets a mind of its own, and it won't stop until you stop it.

"I'll call in your prescription right now," he said.

I drove to CVS, hiccuping the whole way, and picked up the prescription: Thorazine.

I was moving from pot to the hard stuff.

"Take two of these," the pharmacist said, "and you'll be fine."

The prescription was for one hundred pills. As I look back on it, I can say with some degree of certainty that I went home. I must have taken the pills. I honestly can't be sure.

All I know is that I woke up, I don't know how many hours later, slouched in my recliner with the empty IV bottle in my arm.

But I didn't hiccup again.

And if I ever felt the urge to commit an ax murder, I had ninety-eight pills left.

———

I'd been giving myself fluids for a week or two. Whether it was the pot or the passage of time, I started feeling a little better, a little stronger. Parrish, Ash, and his wife, Abisola, needed a break. Even my dogs were sick of me. I told them I was going to the beach—we have a little place in San Simeon. I packed up my IV gear and fluids and drove off.

I resolved to make a concerted effort to eat. I had been getting hunger pangs for the first time again. I'd be watching commercials for Sizzler, or for Outback Steakhouse, or for Jersey Mike's, or Pizza Hut, and I wanted it so bad. The pot may have helped with this. So did another medication called mirtazapine that they give to cancer patients to boost their appetite and make them eat.

I got to the beach, and the munchies returned. Hot damn. I went to the store, and there I saw a can of Progresso minestrone soup. It seemed perfect: soft noodles. I got it home, made it lukewarm so it wouldn't scald my throat, and took one bite, and the salt content and the tomato lit my mouth up.

I lost it. I got really mad. I threw the spoon in the sink. I was by myself, and I just started yelling, "What! The! Fuck!"

I was getting so damn tired of this.

The doctors and the shrink told me that I was going to get angry, that this was one of those good signs, that it was normal. All that resentment would build up and then explode. Let it go, as the song says.

I walked to the sand and looked at the ocean and thought of my grandfather and that day when I told him I was going to Los Angeles. I always remembered his encouragement and how he said he'd break the news to my parents.

"You're going to be in Southern California," he told me. "They call it the Pacific Ocean for a reason. It's peaceful. Throw your cares into the ocean and let it pacify."

I listened to the waves. And he was right.

CHAPTER THIRTEEN

Back to Work, Too Soon

In late June, nearly two months after my last chemotherapy treatment, I called my agent, Cynthia McLean.

"I'm ready to try this," I said.

Cynthia asked if I was sure I could go back to work. I said, "Sure, I'm sure." I promised her I would ease into it. At worst, I would record stuff that would be scratch vocals, placeholder tracks that I could redo later in postproduction.

Cynthia's interest in me goes far beyond her 10 percent. I've had the same agency since I was making fast-food commercials. Cynthia, Rita Vennari, Mary Ellen Lord, and the rest of those incredible human beings at Sutton, Barth & Vennari have been part of my life for forty years.

Cynthia made the calls, which is how I found myself back at the mic. I would leave the house early to give myself plenty of time to make the long drive to Burbank. I would stop at Starbucks near the Nickelodeon studio for a quick calorie-filled Frappuccino, then go to the recording studio.

The producers and other actors on *VeggieTales* and *Teenage Mutant Ninja Turtles* welcomed me back and made every allowance for my health. I tried to do only a few sessions at first, but even a reduced schedule got to me. One morning, after the Starbucks stop, I felt so tired that I pulled over and closed my eyes. I had an hour left before my session was to begin, and it was only a few blocks away. I thought I would catch a minute or two of sleep.

I woke up an hour and a half later, nearly thirty minutes into my session time.

It was long past 11:00 a.m. and I was exhausted, absolutely out of it. I hightailed it over to Nickelodeon, pushed myself up the stairs, and dragged my ass into the studio. I apologized to everyone. The cast and crew and producers couldn't have been nicer. They told me not to worry about it, come in, do my thing.

I did it, but not very well. It was comforting being around creative people again. I wanted to be there because it made my brain happy. But it was a slog. I was weak, exhausted just from driving to Burbank and walking up the stairs to the studio, and I realized I hadn't eaten for a day and a half because I wasn't hungry. I told myself I had to force down a protein shake.

I didn't want to push it. Frankly, I didn't want to screw it up. Any time they told me it seemed like my voice was giving out, I quickly said, "Great, we'll stop."

One day, on *VeggieTales*, they wanted me to do a song in my character. I had done the voices, but this was the first time they wanted me to sing.

The character was, get this, Bacon Bill. It was a piece of talking bacon. I offered to give it my best shot. We could use it as a scratch vocal, and either I or another actor could dub it later. Of course, I'm not used to doing that. I'm used to giving it 100 percent and nailing it, like the first time I did "Yakko's World" in one take. I don't like when I can't do stuff.

I sang in my bacon voice and didn't like it. I didn't have the notes at the top of my range that I used to have, ever since I could remember. I don't mean just Hollywood. I mean way, way, way back in Michigan, when I was singing for Sass. And those notes are important, because they make me the singer I am. To miss them was really rough.

I told myself, *Give yourself a break. That's just today. Remember what you've gone through. You're back working. Let's consider this a win for today, something to hold on to when you close your eyes and go to sleep. There's always time for another go.*

One man at DreamWorks on this *VeggieTales* project came up to me on his own, without the other folks around. He took a moment to say, "I just wanna tell you how much I appreciate you being here and also, I just want to tell you that I get your struggle."

"What?" I asked. "Did you have throat cancer?"

"No, I had prostate cancer. But it was tough."

"Oh man," I said. "Are you okay?"

"Yeah, I'm good," he said. "It took me about a year and a half to get my shit together. It was a lot of radiation and all that."

But he said, "For me, it was about being tired and exhausted. I didn't have the pain. In fact, in my case, I don't recall having a lot of discomfort. I was getting treatment with a guy I got to know who was having your treatment. And he said it was brutal."

"It's not a question of degrees," I said. "It's a question of we're both kind of kindred spirits."

He nodded. "If you ever want to talk, if you ever want to discuss it, I'm here."

Once someone finds out you're in the same club that neither of you want to be a member of, you're both inextricably linked forever. It felt like this was somebody with whom I could be completely honest and, if I got to a place where I wanted to say, "I don't like this. I don't like feeling this way, but right now, I am so disgusted with my life. I'm so angry that I can't taste a piece of chocolate cake, or that I can't eat a piece of fish, or that I can't have a cocktail," that person wouldn't judge me.

I was finally willing to have somebody be a hero to me. It could be for just a few minutes—somebody could do something that I needed right there. They didn't ask anything in return. I needed them. I learned to be vulnerable.

I needed to be able to let my guard down and not be Mr. Happy all the time. I found that there were times, now, when I couldn't muster the strength to amuse other people. I didn't want to muster that strength. Knowing that there were people who understood what I was going through was a big step for me.

I got what it's like to feel truly awful. And I finally realized: it's not all about me helping them. It's about them helping me. Moreover, me allowing them to. When, as an adult, you can allow yourself to be vulnerable, it really does, I think, enable you to be more human. It opened up a side of me that often I would protect because I didn't want to seem weak, or I didn't want to seem unhappy. Or I didn't want to seem ungrateful.

It turns out that part of being human is being able to let people see the not-so-pleasant sides of yourself. That is a skill I'm still learning. Knowing, really knowing, that there are people who are willing to listen to you and talk about how miserable you are raises my game at every level.

A few days later, I was home by myself on my computer listening to iTunes on the speakers in the house. I had a Kenny Loggins record on, *Celebrate Me Home*, which was one of the seminal records of my twenties. I was always a Loggins and Messina fan. Kenny Loggins is a terrific singer, right in my wheelhouse. I auditioned with Kenny Loggins songs to get jobs when I first got to Hollywood. I could sing like that. That was my vibe.

I was sitting there humming along with Kenny on my computer, by myself, with just my Yorkies, Tala and Pooshie, for company, when I realized that I was singing along with the record. I was hitting most of the notes. It wasn't perfect. But it was way better than it had been.

I got pretty shaken up, in a good way. I had to catch myself. I was getting tearful. I thought, *That's it. I'm actually able to do this.*

It was one of those small victories. With cancer, you come to treasure the tiniest of wins. When I found myself singing along with a Kenny Loggins record that I used to audition with in the late '70s, that was important. Here I was, sixty years old, and that alone was a big deal—to be able to sing those songs at sixty. But to be able to hit those notes after throat cancer and know that, "Okay, it might be a while, but I'm gonna get them back"? That was definitely a victory.

I went back to the studio for another round with Bacon Bill's song, telling myself, *I'm not going to freak out.*

As it turned out, they only had a few pickups that they wanted me to do, just two parts of the song that didn't sound right. That song I thought I had butchered? Eighty percent of it was where it needed to be.

My perception of how good or bad I was had become completely skewed. The voice lesson was: my best is sometimes good enough. Is it perfect? No. Is it where you'd like it to be? No. But it's enough.

To want what you have and to take what you're given—that is where the grace of embracing horrible circumstances comes in, whether it's cancer, losing a loved one, a car accident, or your house burning down. Getting through it is about letting go and understanding that there are people who can make some judgments better than you. You do your best and you go ahead and you move on. It's okay not to be perfect. It's okay to be good enough.

I wondered if this is what Chad's family went through. They weren't going to make him perfect again, not by a long shot. They were going to lose him, at a young age. Yet they persisted. That was all they could do. Their best was the best that could be done, and judging themselves too harshly served no purpose. They could let other people call them heroes, people like me.

Even if on their worst days that wasn't entirely true, it was true enough.

In July of 2016, Nickelodeon asked if I would do some promotional stuff for the new *Teenage Mutant Ninja Turtles* series at Comic-Con in San Diego. The studio wanted to send the entire new cast.

Then I got a call from Sam Register at Warner Bros. We had kept in touch since the dinner meeting. He said the studio was able to get a room on the last day of Comic-Con, I think at around three o'clock that Sunday afternoon, and they wanted to bring down the cast of *Animaniacs*, all of us—Tress, Jess, Maurice, and Randy.

The studio and Mr. Spielberg had still not made a decision on the reboot. Like the live shows Randy and I did, this looked to be another trial balloon, to see how the audience reacted to the old gang, see if there even was an audience. Warner Bros. had high hopes; the hall sat a thousand people.

I can't be sure, but I think it was also a test for me. I had been back to work. But could I do it at the highest level? Could I not only pull off the voices, but could I still sing? And would it sound like it did twenty years ago?

I said yes to both Nickelodeon and Warner Bros. I said I'd drive myself to San Diego. I like cars. I like to drive. The doctors didn't object. They just told me to make sure to slather myself in Purell because my immune system had taken a hit, like it does with any cancer patient. They didn't want me coming back from San Diego with dengue fever.

I wanted to jump back into the mix. I'd already had these moments where I was getting my shit together, and this was an opportunity to take it to the next level, to do music in front of people, with my friends, and a chance to see if I could really pull it off.

I savored the challenge, but I think I was also just proving to myself that I was bigger than the cancer, that I was stronger than the debilitating treatment. It really kicked my ass, and I needed to know that I could do my work again.

The biggest roadblock to this plan was my wife. She really didn't want me to go. And she didn't want me driving.

I pushed. She pushed back harder. I think my wife's reasoning was sound. My reasoning was more emotional.

Without telling me, she called my agent and told her she didn't want me driving to San Diego. She asked if Nickelodeon could split the cost of a car service.

I was a little bit taken aback when I found out my agent and my wife had conspired behind my back to get me this ride down there. But we found a trade-off. The agreement with my wife was that she'd be okay with me going down if I got a ride. She was right. It was a much better way to go. Nickelodeon jumped right up to it, and they got me a town car. I definitely was not 100 percent, and she knew it. I was too tired to have driven all that way. I was living on venti caramel Frappuccinos with no whipped cream. It's five hundred useless calories, but for whatever reason, that was one of the only things I could taste a little bit.

When I got to the hotel in San Diego, somebody from Nickelodeon offered me a sandwich. I took two bites and couldn't get it down. I didn't throw it up; I just couldn't swallow it. Salads were the same way. Not only did food lack taste, I physically couldn't get it down my throat. It was the result of having at least a couple of my salivary glands obliterated.

I was able to eat soups by this point. I remember having lunch on the hotel veranda. Randy and I were out there with his sister, who's from San Diego. I ordered a bowl of tomato bisque, and I got it all down.

"Good for you, buddy," Randy said.

The plan was to sign autographs and do a panel for Nickelodeon on the new *Turtles*. I had started recording that in March of 2011, and it had premiered in September of 2012 with the new cast: Leonardo was Jason Biggs, I was Donatello, Raphael was Sean Astin, Michelangelo was Greg Cipes, and Master Splinter was an incredible actor named Hoon Lee. Shredder, the bad guy, was Kevin Michael Richardson.

Then I was free to hang out for the weekend, relax, and then do the *Animaniacs* event with Randy and Tress and Jess on Sunday. I wasn't sure how many people would actually attend. We got down there, and the place was overflowing with fans. The fire marshal had to turn a few hundred people away. We filled up the thousand-seat room, even though the con was almost over and a lot of people were already on their way home. Our fans stuck around to see us and hear the music.

I hadn't made any announcement about my treatment. It seemed, at my standing in Hollywood, presumptuous to even think of it. I wasn't expecting the world to stop and say, "Oh my God." I wasn't like Michael Douglas, who had people taking his picture walking in and out of the clinic and asking, *why is he so skinny?*

At Comic-Con, however, people *were* taking pictures of me. I was down to about 130 pounds. "Why are you so thin? Are you okay?" the fans asked. They wanted to know what happened to my podcast. So I started telling people as discreetly as possible about my cancer. It wasn't a big announcement, but I let people know, one by one.

I had some inkling that this would be the beginning of me setting an example. During my treatment, I met people going through their second or third time in the cancer cage getting chemo and radiation. They often looked almost like skeletons, and they were going out, finding ways to live their lives. They were walking from cancer chair to cancer chair to see if they could get me anything. "Hey, Rob, you want some water?"

This appearance at Comic-Con was going to be the beginning of me saying, "Well, I'm not 100 percent, but I'm out here doing it." I did look really skinny. My eyes had kind of a sunken look, and I seemed like I was a little bit lost. But I hoped that when people found out what the reasoning was and what the story was with me, why I had dragged my skinny ass out there, wearing my size-29 jeans, maybe somebody would be a little bit inspired, like I had been inspired by so many others.

We did about ten songs together and separately on the *Animaniacs* panel. My voice was maybe 75 percent. My breakthrough with Bacon Bill notwithstanding, I still had to change the melodies of some of the higher-pitched songs to accommodate my more limited range. I figured, hey, other singers do it. Elton John has done it for years and nobody gives a shit, with one minor but significant difference: he's Elton John.

I felt that it was only about being true to the music. It would be better to change a few things than to hit clunkers and try to explain myself later. I remembered the voice lesson—it was not about being perfect, it was about being enough. When you're able to give yourself the freedom to be enough, it's pretty sweet.

The hardest song was "Yakko's World." I was supposed to sing it live with Randy at the electric piano. It was a little difficult, because when you start to get nervous, your mouth gets dry anyway. Now, when your mouth gets dry *and* you have no saliva glands, like me, it's like someone doing a production of *Lawrence of Arabia* in your mouth. (I would submit that it probably tasted like camels walking through my mouth, too, because one of the cool things about saliva is it helps you with things like bad breath. I don't think anybody went out of their way to tell me my breath stunk, but it was really harrowing.)

Then, of course, the dryness extends to your throat. I probably went through three bottles of water onstage. I would drink during songs, between bridges. I told Randy to keep "Yakko's World" in the key in which we started. When you listen to the song, it goes up a half step, four times. So by the time that I sing the last verse, it's two full steps up from the original note I started on. That's the way it was recorded, and that's the way I do it now. But when I did it at Comic-Con that day, we kept it in the same key.

And it didn't matter one bit to the audience. They got on their feet and applauded. There were a number of wet eyes in the house, not the least of which was mine.

I scanned the audience, and I had personal friends who had stuck around, who knew what was going on. Townsend Coleman, one of the original Turtles, one of the guys I had to call when I canceled out on the conventions, had tears in his eyes.

It was something I'd done hundreds of times, but this was, incredibly, the first time again. Completely different. It was the beginning of Rob 2.0, as one of my friends has called me. I would have much bigger gigs a few months later, but for now, I was back in the mix.

The whole weekend, my wife was checking in on me and was very concerned. I told her I was okay. I didn't lose my voice. Nothing hurt any worse. I was pretty exhausted, but I didn't have to go to work the next day, on Monday.

On the ride back that Sunday, I slept in the car.

The reality was I shouldn't have gone back so quickly. I was scary thin. I couldn't handle solid food. My salivary glands had been torched by the radiation, so my throat suffered from chronic dryness. I drank lots of water. Rather than listening to my body, I was trying to make a point to myself.

Before cancer, I had been as healthy as a horse. The worst that had ever happened was I'd gotten my nose broken and a few teeth chipped playing hockey. I had never been involved in anything that I couldn't handle. I had never felt like I lost so much control before, and now it was twenty-five or thirty minutes of uncontrollable dry heaving, or falling asleep in the middle of the day. I wanted to get myself back to some semblance of normalcy.

Nobody wants a second shot at cancer. If you're fortunate, you only have to go one round with the disease. (If you're extremely fortunate, you don't even have to do that.) So it's odd in some ways to think about what I would do differently if I had to do cancer over again. But that's what passed through my mind.

If I had to do it over again, I would find a different way of making myself feel more in control. It seemed so important at the time that I pushed myself too hard. It wasn't just returning to work prematurely. I remember going to the gym and telling the trainer that I lost a lot of weight but that I wanted to get back in shape. Two minutes on the stationary bike and I was ready to puke. I get exhausted just thinking about it.

If I had to do it all over again, I maybe would just take walks, something a little less onerous. I get why I leaped back into work. So much of who I am is about my ability to do my gig, not for the money, but to make people laugh and to entertain myself, to come up with a character or a voice and to be able to do all this at the highest level. You don't know if you can handle it until you get back to work. I wanted to get back into the fight, as it were. It was my fight. But I had to learn to deal with the compromises. If I had to do it over again, I would understand from the outset that sometimes it doesn't have to be perfect. It has to be enough.

I should have listened better. I should have listened to my wife.

Losing control to cancer touches something primal. You're a hunter-gatherer, stuck back in the cave, watching somebody else feed your family. It attacks more than just your physicality. It hits you where you live.

I remember when my father had gotten to the point where we had to take the car keys from him. He had become a danger to himself and everyone else in northern Michigan. I got a call from him every day after that, reminding me that his oldest child took away his car keys.

I kept reliving that depressing time a few years earlier, when work got slow and I panicked. And I thought about it frequently now as I tried to swallow food each day.

What I had to realize was that I'd lost control incrementally, and that's how I would have to get it back. It's about balance. It's about taking a breath. It's about living that moment.

CHAPTER FOURTEEN

Throat Flambé

After Comic-Con, I had another PET scan. This was the same test that found the tumor, the one that lit up like a Christmas tree. The doctors on my team huddled together and said the scan looked good. There was just a little bit of a hot spot in my throat, but this soon after treatment, that wasn't unusual. It could be inflammation.

It was full speed ahead. No more treatments. I'd have another PET scan in three months.

Then I got a call from one of my doctors.

"I go to bed every night worried about my patients," he told me. "I'd really like you to do that biopsy again. Just to make sure. It's probably an 85 percent chance that the hot spot isn't cancer. But if it comes back and we didn't get it, then you have a problem. We want to be 100 percent sure."

It took me about ten seconds before I said, "Wow, okay."

I was on the mend. I still couldn't taste, but I was starting to gain weight. I was up about eight pounds.

I thought about how much the original biopsy hurt. I shuddered at what that would feel like on raw, radiated skin.

I called my wife, and she lost it. "Are you fucking kidding me?" She thought it was an overreaction, that the doctor was being an alarmist, that another biopsy would set back my recovery for weeks, maybe months.

"I've got to do it, honey," I said. "He's the boss."

I polled the other doctors, and I sensed a subtle shift. Those who'd seemed firm in their convictions that I should stay the course and skip the biopsy had begun to waver. When I pressed them, they said things like, "I understand. You have to do what's best."

I have to? This potentially life-or-death medical decision rests with a college dropout who makes his living as singing bacon?

I get it. We live in such a litigious society. Nobody wants to get sued. If one doctor says, "I don't care what the other doctor says, don't get that biopsy," and then the patient drops dead, guess who's getting dragged into court.

It was a jumble of messages. On the one hand, I was warned not to rush to the internet for second opinions, because I would get misinformation. On the other hand, what was I supposed to base my decision on? I was caught between a rock and a hard place, and that rock might be my tombstone.

If I looked at it from a percentage point of view, I had four out of five doctors recommending against the biopsy. That's fine for buying toothpaste, but no way to make a life-or-death decision. If the cancer does come back, it's bad. Super bad. They really start cutting you up, taking pieces out of your face.

I bit the bullet.

"All right," I told my doctor. "I can handle this."

When I had the first biopsy, I was all gung-ho and joking with the nurses and of course talking in the voices once they found out who I was. It was fun. I liked the attention. And it seemed to make everybody happy. Here we go. Bring on the pain medication! Woo hoo. I like Vicodin, anyway. How bad can it be?

It was different this time around. After my wife and son drove me to the clinic for the second biopsy, one of the nurses recognized me and said, "Oh, you're back. Everything okay?"

I mumbled, "Yeah."

They weighed me on the bed. I didn't even know they could weigh you on the bed. I was 134 pounds. Lighter than I even thought. For a guy who is five nine and a half and a medium/average build, that meant I'd lost 30 percent of my body weight.

I remembered what Randy had told me during the most difficult times of chemotherapy. This West Point grad offered advice from a military point of view. When things got bad, he said, "Put your head down and take that hill."

I was definitely not the effusive funny guy from the first biopsy. No jokes, no silly voices, no bantering with the nurses, no trying to make the other patients happy. It was all about getting through this.

They knocked me out and did the procedure while I was under. When I woke up, the pain was, to use a medical term, a real motherfucker. The first biopsy hurt. This was hurt on top of hurt.

After a recovery period in the clinic, I somehow got to the car. I don't remember much. I'm sure Ash had to help me. The doctor had said pathology would provide the final word, but he thought everything was going to be fine.

As we pulled away, my wife said, "I'm so glad, and fuck that doctor."

She was still steaming, and no surprise. She had another month or two of me hooked up to an IV in the TV room, sleeping and shrinking.

My wife said, "Would you like a Malibu Dream, honey?"

Along with Starbucks Frappuccinos, my go-to drink was a frozen slushy drink called a Malibu Dream at Coffee Bean.

"Boy, that sounds great," I said.

We got to the Coffee Bean. I was a little bit drowsy. I took a sip, and my throat ignited. I didn't yell. I didn't scream. I didn't say anything. I just put the straw down. And then my son looked at me and said, "Are you okay, Dad?"

"I just can't drink it," I said quietly.

With cancer, you gauge courage and strength in tiny increments. I didn't need to be Superman just then. I just had to deal with what was happening right now, take that hill and worry about the other ones later.

I had tried to put on a brave face for my son throughout my treatments. When I finished radiation, we posed for a selfie, both with big smiles. It's one of my favorite photos of the two of us. I never wanted my son to know how frightened I was.

Now there was no hiding anything. It reminded me of when I saw my own father, in 2005, as he recovered from quadruple bypass surgery in the hospital in Michigan. He woke up and asked me to shave him. He wanted to be more presentable for the rest of the family. I had never seen my father incapacitated before—he had always been strong and intimidating. Now he was gray, in hair and face. He was an old, sick man.

That's how I felt after that second biopsy. I was twenty years younger than my father had been when he was in the hospital, but I was just as helpless, suffering just as much pain. It was a stark reminder of my own mortality. But as awful as I looked and felt, I was actually glad my son could see me this way. I was vulnerable. I needed his help, and he gave it. He has always been a source of pride and strength to me.

For the next few weeks, I don't know if I was depressed, but it definitely felt like a setback. It was really painful. It took a long time to heal. I stopped eating again. I lost what little weight I'd gained. I was back to just mainly swallowing, if I could, water. I was back to getting no nutrition.

I cursed my doctor for not insisting on getting the feeding tube. My wife was incredibly angry.

It wasn't like I was suicidal. It was just: this is really getting to be a problem.

I would have moments when I really got frustrated, and then I'd smack myself: dude, just take a breath. Go suck on an Ensure, hook yourself up to fluids, take your Vicodin, watch a hockey game.

And think about Chad.

One day, his mother called me. "You have to hear this."

I said, "What, what?"

"Well, Chad is finally strong enough to go in and have a surgical procedure in which the doctors are able to install two stainless steel rods on either side of his spine, to help him sit more upright. That'll really alleviate the mucus issues in his lungs."

Which is often what kills people in his circumstance. So it would give him a better quality life and a longer life. He hadn't been strong enough to go through that surgery before.

"Here's the kicker," she said. "The only way he would get the surgery done was if the doctors allowed him to wear his Turtle jacket."

She said he was adamant: "I won't let you do this surgery unless I wear this Turtle jacket." And he was, I dunno, nine?

The doctors got together with his mother and father, and they talked about it and said, "All right, Chad, here's the deal, what we'll do is—so you understand—we have to operate on your back. And, if you were wearing a jacket, we might mess up your jacket. You've got the only Ninja Turtle Raphael jacket in the universe. So, what we'll do is, we'll sterilize the jacket, put it in a plastic bag, and we'll drape it over you as we go into surgery. And when you wake up, it will be on you, okay?"

And he said, "Okay."

They made a deal with him. He had the surgery, came through it, got to use his jacket, all of that.

It was another moment that sort of dropped me to my emotional knees.

He had to live his life. His parents had to live every day, one day at a time. They had to take a moment to step outside and go, "Whoo. Okay. Here we go." And then go back inside. Because they knew nothing different—that was their reality.

I do know something different. But I had to live, right now, in this moment, and deal with this pain or this disappointment right now. I had to face one hill at a time.

They were doing the same thing I was, and I didn't realize it. What other option did they have but to deal with the issues before them now and not think too hard about the future, because that could drive them insane? What other options did I have than to just bumble through?

So just right now, this pain from the biopsy is a problem, I told myself. *Maybe tomorrow it'll be a problem. Let's just not freak out.* And that was a conscious choice. I really started living in the moment, dealing with problems as they arose, and not projecting a month down the road or two months down the road, making me and everybody else miserable.

After a while, Chad and I lost touch. Years went by and I didn't hear from his family, and didn't want to invade their privacy to find out what was going on. Then one day around 2007 or 2008, I went on MySpace—you remember MySpace?—and out of the blue, I got a message from Chad.

I said, "Oh my god, Chad! How are ya, buddy?"

He was in his early twenties. He had made it long past the age most kids in his condition do.

"I'm good, man," he said. He showed me a picture of himself. He was obviously still in the wheelchair, but otherwise I barely recognized him. He had grown a goatee and had gotten tattoos. And, he said, "I still got my Turtle jacket."

"Thank God," I said. "It's great to hear from you."

We exchanged information and got back into talking to each other via social media. Then I was going to Canada for my first animation convention, called Calgary Expo: Comics & Entertainment.

I told his sister Jennifer, the oldest one who did not have MD, "Jen, I would love to see you guys. Is there any way you can get Chad there?"

There was a five-hundred-seat theater at the Expo in which Jess and I were giving a little Q&A, doing a panel discussion about our work. Someone in the audience asked, "What's the coolest thing about being a voice actor?"

I looked out of the corner of my eye, and there was Chad, on a walkway, next to where everybody was sitting. I started to choke up.

"You know what the coolest thing about this gig is?" And I started telling the story about Chad, a truncated version. Then I said, "And the gentleman that I'm talking about is right over there."

Jen brought him up, and everybody stood, and it was unbelievable. It was like *Mr. Holland's Opus.* I just went over there and I put my arms around him. He was thin, frail, covered in tattoos but living his life, man.

It was really a remarkable experience. I had this gift of being able to show this audience what Turtle power was all about. Honest to Christ, Turtle power. And that's exactly what it was.

Chad lived to be twenty-five. That's a pretty long time for a kid with Duchenne muscular dystrophy. When it was his time, his mother sent me a Facebook message.

"You'll never know what you meant to my son," she said.

It was really the other way around. That indelible mark that Chad and his family left on my soul and my heart is a far greater gift than what I gave to Chad.

"No," I said, "you'll never know what he meant to me."

All this came flooding back when I would start to go into my dark little places. I had already beaten the odds. I had already made it to sixty years old. My throat was going to hurt a little bit; I was going to lose a bit of weight. But when I was done, I would have a great story to tell and maybe I'd be able to help other people.

The first biopsy took two weeks to heal. This one took six weeks. But the bottom line was: the treatment worked. The lump in my neck was gone. I mean, it was gone. It was remarkable seeing it shrink while the radiation was doing its thing. The best possible outcome was realized. I knew that I didn't have to go through the chemo and radiation again.

There was a price to pay, and I paid it. The doctor gave me peace of mind with that second biopsy, so kudos to him.

Then I got a new doctor.

CHAPTER FIFTEEN

Faith, Kindness, Passion, Humor . . . and Cheez-Its

By the end of 2016 and early 2017, I experienced another milestone: I could eat Cheez-Its again.

Before my cancer treatment, these orange crackers had been my favorite guilty pleasure. Once the radiation started, they were the first to go. Where I used to enjoy Cheez-Its by the handful, now it was like chewing on ping-pong balls and sand. They just stuck in my throat. If I wasn't careful, I could aspirate and choke.

That's not the way I wanted to go. I'd rather die, like, in a fire trying to save a dog or a valuable painting. I could picture the obit: he was a really good guy, a funny guy, and get this . . . he died choking on Cheez-Its.

The scar tissue narrowed my esophagus. It has not affected my ability to do my job, but it affects the way I consume food. If I take a big bite of something, it gets stuck. I've been told there's a procedure to stretch out my esophagus. You need general anesthesia, because obviously if they start shoving shit down your throat, it makes you gag. So they put a little device down there that stretches it out. It would probably break some adhesions and bleed a little bit.

If I can avoid that, I will.

I'm very careful now. I snap the Cheez-It into more manageable bites, the way a parent cuts food for a baby. They can now get down my scarred throat. Small victories.

In 2017, I was feeling so much better that I began to book conventions again, the first time since that exhausting Comic-Con six months earlier. The first booked show was one of my favorites, the Marvelous Nerd Year's Eve convention in Dallas during the first weekend of 2017. Tress, Jess, Maurice, and I attended. Moe and I got to roast the legendary Stan Lee onstage with Michael Rooker from *The Walking Dead* and Ming-Na Wen from *Agents of S.H.I.E.L.D.*

I was still very thin, very tired, but very grateful and *very* excited to be back with fans. I was signing autographs when this tall, husky guy came up. In my Pinky voice, I said, "You're a big one, aren't you?"

And then he cried.

He composed himself and explained that he was a veteran, and he talked about how he used to take his *Pinky and the Brain*, *Animaniacs*, and *Batman* DVDs with him on deployments to Iraq and Afghanistan. He'd come back from an operation, pop a DVD in, and take his mind off everything. I tried to wrap my head around it. My job requires me to be funny. His job required him to not get killed.

For a little while, this big soldier could be ten years old again and at home, curled up in front of the television, safe from the world. I thought of the miracles that are these characters, how, yes, they can bring you a smile and a laugh, but also so much more.

The next morning, in my hotel room, I was in a reflective mood. I got out a microphone, hooked it into my iPad, and spoke slowly.

"Faith, kindness, passion, humor. Oh, and Cheez-Its. Those five things are what anybody needs in their life to be happy, as far as I'm concerned. That's certainly what I needed in my life," I said. "Hi, it's Rob Paulsen, and I'm back."

More than a year had passed since I'd last recorded a podcast. It was time to start anew, time to officially go public. I thanked my fans for their patience. "It's clear that you have a love for the podcast that is beyond anything I could have hoped for, which shows me how much smarter you guys are than me," I said. "I'm here to explain the whole shooting match. Rob explains it all today."

I recounted how I was diagnosed with throat cancer after finding the lump. "As you can imagine, that really got my attention," I said. "Trust me, the twisted irony of a guy making a living with his voice being diagnosed with throat cancer was not lost on me."

I explained how I was told that I'd survive with treatment, but that the cancer would kick my ass, which was why I had been out of commission for so long. And I came clean about the story about the nodes.

"I lied," I said. "I'm fessing up a bit. I lied because I didn't want people to freak out. I didn't need sympathy. I don't want sympathy. The day I got my phone call confirming my diagnosis, thousands of other people just in LA were getting the same phone call, and often about their four- or five-year-old. God forbid, can you imagine—and people deal with that all the time. And I did not have to.

"Look, you guys, I am sixty years old. And even if they had said to me, here's the deal, man, you better get your stuff in order because you're on your way out, we're getting ready to punch your ticket, I've had a hell of a life and an incredible career, a wonderful run, a terrific childhood. Parrish, my wife, has been unbelievably heroic through this whole thing. I had great doctors. I have nothing to feel sorry about. Please don't shed a tear for me."

For those who would meet me or see pictures of me, I explained that through the radiation and chemotherapy I had lost about fifty pounds. But now I was recording my podcast again, going to conventions, recording character voices for shows.

"I'm getting my shit together, baby. I'm ready to rock and roll," I said. "I did have cancer. I do not, anymore, according to my doctors. So now I have this gift, as a result of my cancer treatment. I now believe I have a more interesting story to tell, and I have a more helpful story to tell."

It was a relief to come clean. I realize I wasn't the nightly focus of *Entertainment Tonight*. But ever since Comic-Con, people had been asking what was wrong with me, why I was so skinny. It felt good to get this off my chest and be real clear to people that not only was I okay, but I would have a happy ending, that I was starting a new chapter in my life.

One day back in 2016, while I was starting my recovery, I spoke to my brother, Mike. He was an actor for many years in New York. He's semiretired now and works for Broadway Cares three days a week.

Earlier in the year, while I was in the midst of my radiation and chemo, he had told me about a very close friend, an actor he'd known for years, who had the same type of cancer that I did. The doctors were concerned because the friend was one hundred pounds overweight with diabetic issues.

"Yeah, man, this is brutal," I said at the time. "I know what he's fixing to go through. If he wants a sensitive ear, please don't hesitate. And you know that I'm serious, Mike."

He said, yeah, no problem.

I never heard from the guy. A few months later, when I was getting back on my feet, I asked Mike, "By the way, how's your buddy hanging in?"

He kind of stopped. "He didn't make it."

I said, "Holy fuck, really?"

"They went in and they gave him the treatment that you had, they gave him a food tube, all that stuff. The cancer and the treatment were too intense for his compromised state."

I felt like I'd received a gut punch. I didn't even know this guy. Then I realized I did: he could have been me.

This was somebody my brother had spoken about many times for twenty-odd years. His diagnosis was the same as mine. And he died.

My brother said, "I didn't tell you because I didn't want to upset you."

I said, "No, no, I totally understand."

It brought it home. Maybe for the first time, I realized: you can really die from this. Somehow hearing about somebody else's experience made mine more real. This guy didn't make it.

I had to hang up the phone and take a breath.

Somebody, somewhere, was telling a person they love, "I've got cancer," or "It's back," or "It's stage V, and it's in my liver." It wasn't me this time, but it could have been.

I've learned life cries wolf a lot. And most of the time, the wolf isn't at the door. There's a lot of shit we can get upset about, and it's often our perspective that's really the problem.

I recorded another podcast a month later, a Reddit AMA—Ask Me Anything—fielding questions in real time from my house. A month after that I sat down in a studio with Christian Lanz, best known for doing voices on the TV series *Elena of Avalor* and a bunch of video games like the *Call of Duty* series and various *Batman* games. We had worked together on the new *Turtles* series. Next I interviewed Caitlin Glass, a wonderful voice actress who works in anime shows.

The podcast got me back in the saddle, helping me become more self-sufficient. I could make my own work, hire myself. It was a wonderful way to interact with fans. The audience kept building. And one day, after all these years, it finally turned a buck.

Nerdist picked up *Talkin' Toons* and installed me in a high-tech studio with four HD cameras, and now the show streams as audio and video. They promoted the hell out of it. I even got my own billboard on La Cienega, a towering cartoon version of me smiling down on the people stuck in traffic.

It was like gasoline pouring on my creative fire. I reached out to Randy about restarting our live performances. We wanted to make a big splash. In April 2017, in the LA suburb of La Mirada, less than an hour down the freeway from the animation studios, we had our most ambitious show ever: two two-hour shows, back to back, featuring twenty songs, covering the best and zaniest from *Animaniacs*, featuring not only Randy and me, but also Tress and Jess.

We'd be accompanied by the forty-four-piece La Mirada Symphony Orchestra, giving the songs the same lush, professional, top-notch musical quality that set *Animaniacs* ahead of the cartoon pack. The shows sold out the La Mirada Theatre, a total of twenty-four hundred tickets.

This would be our first truly local crowd: friends, family, colleagues, and a number of executives from Warner Bros. If the Comic-Con show the previous July was meant to see if anybody was still interested in *Animaniacs*, this program seemed designed to help the executives make up their minds. I'd be kidding myself if I said I didn't think the executives came in part just to see if I still had anything left in the tank.

I thought the Comic-Con gig went well, all things considered. But that was at a comic convention, where the audience could have just meandered into the room looking for the snack bar and wound up listening to me. The La Mirada show was by far the biggest paying audience we'd had, and the nerves hit me again. The more nervous I got, the more my mouth went dry. I brought three bottles of water onstage.

This night, the stakes were much higher. It was my first big live performance since the cancer diagnosis: April 15, 2017. Tax day. Failure would drop me into the zero bracket.

I wore a purple shirt I had purchased when I was about forty-five pounds heavier. It fit me like a caftan. I looked like I had bought my clothes at Redondo Beach Tent and Awning instead of Hugo Boss. I hadn't gotten any new clothes because I thought I was going to gain the weight back. I didn't, and I looked like shit.

Despite outward appearances, I felt pretty good physically. My voice had gotten stronger. I sang in the car the day before the show and was able to hit the higher notes. And even if I couldn't, so what? I'm not Pavarotti, I'm a cartoon singer. But because of the scar tissue in my throat, my esophagus and trachea would still constrict. For that I drank lots of water.

Just before the first performance, I closed my eyes. I kept reminding myself of how long it had taken and how hard it was to get to this point, how in my darkest moments I feared I would never be able to talk again, much less sing for an audience.

I walked out from stage right and hit my mark downstage front center. The first thing I did was look over to Randy at the piano. He calms me down. I'm out there with a world-class performer, knowing that if I go absolutely into the dumper, Randy will pick it up. Although there's a narrative arc to *Animaniacs Live!*, there's an extemporaneous element to the show that the audience likes. We kind of go from song to song with an idea of what we're going to say in between, but it changes every time.

Over the years, I'm sure he's glanced at me more than once, when I looked like a frozen steer, and said, "Okay, here's what's next," moving us on to the next song. Randy's my security blanket, albeit one in a nice sport coat and Italian shoes.

During the show, I love seeing the audience. I pick out somebody with green hair or an *Animaniacs* hat and play with them. But as I stood there that night in La Mirada, I was blinded by the stage lights. All I could see was the glare. There's something pretty cool about not being able to see the audience.

"Hellooooo, La Mirada!" Randy and I began.

And the audience lost its mind. Total ape shit. Crazy. The applause washed over me and filled me up and gave me life. It was a transcendent experience.

I took a lot of great drugs during cancer treatment. Nothing compared to this.

The orchestra hit the first note. I cleared my throat—my bruised and battered, poked and chemically fried throat, the source of so much joy and so much pain. I allowed myself one last moment for doubt: *Oh my God, am I ready for this?*

It was time to jump into the deep end, time to sing a silly song.

That whole experience, from conception to execution, was a roller coaster, and as we got to the end of the first act, it was like hurtling down Splash Mountain, just a pure, unadulterated thrill ride. We sent the audience into intermission with the original "Yakko's World," the conductor leading the orchestra, the cartoon running on the screen over my head, and me soaring on autopilot. The music and the character took hold of me and carried me through. Those notes I couldn't hit at Comic-Con had returned like old friends, and I was hitting the higher register again. With each verse, I felt stronger.

The song ended, and the audience cheered. Once again, Yakko saved me.

The bookings for *Animaniacs Live!* poured in: San Francisco; Chicago; Danbury, Connecticut; Honolulu; Atlanta; St. Paul, Minnesota; Oklahoma City; and eight dates at Joe's Pub in Manhattan, publicized with a light-up advertisement in Times frickin' Square. We paid back our investors. We paid back ourselves. We got into the black and built up a chunk of dough to reinvest in the show. We even have our own company now, R&R Productions, for Rob and Randy.

Way back, a lifetime ago, at that dinner in 2016, Sam Register had told us we were on Steven time, and he wasn't kidding. We thought it would be in the next several months that we would hear something. That turned out not to be the case.

We'd check in from time to time, and he would say, "Things look good. They're moving forward. Hang in there."

The following year, 2017, he was telling us, "Okay. Steven's on board. He's going to the pitches." That meant meetings between him and the networks, which included Hulu, Netflix, Apple, and Amazon. I was just awfully, beautifully surprised, wonderfully surprised, that Steven himself was pitching the show.

Streaming appeared to be the best fit for *Animaniacs*. Netflix for, I guess, about a year or so had streamed reruns, and it had done very well for a show that hadn't made a new episode in twenty years. I was quite familiar with how popular it was getting.

Then, in May of 2017, a couple weeks after the La Mirada show, Sam said, "Okay, the pitches are complete, and now we kind of wait and see who wants to do it."

We literally thought it would be within the next week or two, any day now. Instead, weeks, then months went by.

Randy and I were on the road with *Animaniacs Live!*, working clubs and small theaters, just Randy on the piano and me with the voices. The crowds loved the shows, but still radio silence from Mr. Spielberg and Warner Bros.

By October 2017, I was heading to New York Comic-Con, and I was getting worried because we hadn't heard anything about *Animaniacs*. I began to convince myself that the reason I hadn't heard anything was because they were going to cast someone in my place and Sam didn't know how to break it to me. I thought, *You know, it would not surprise me if they're going to replace us with celebrities*. Because it happens.

So there's the insecurity and the ego again—a) that I thought Sam would be thinking about me, and b) that because it was slow, and because it takes a while—even though this is not unusual, it's Steven Spielberg—I automatically assumed I was fired.

I got so worked up I sent Sam a text as I was boarding a plane to go to the convention: "Look, Sam, you have been so fantastic through this whole thing, and I just want you to know that whether they use us or not, I am so grateful that you've been . . . You've been instrumental in *Animaniacs Live!* You were incredibly helpful in helping Randy and me get our licensing deals, so anything above that is gravy."

Within five minutes I got a text from Sam going, "What are you talking about? What happened?"

It was kind of embarrassing, but also reassuring because I hadn't heard, and I hadn't heard, and we had hoped that we maybe could make some announcement at New York Comic-Con. But, Sam assured me, "Nobody's replacing anybody."

It just was taking a while.

After arriving in New York, I was getting ready to go to have dinner in Manhattan, and I got a text from Sam saying, "Okay." This is on a Friday. "Okay, next Tuesday we're going to let people know."

I said, "Okey dokey." And I went back and I mentioned it to Randy, who was there because we were doing our first gig at Joe's Pub.

I said, "Hey, I think we're going to make the announcement on Tuesday, and keep your eye on the internet and HollywoodReporter. com, whatever."

Tuesday came and went. Crickets. That went on for months. It wasn't until the beginning of 2018 that an announcement came out.

I saw it on the *Hollywood Reporter's* website on January 4: *'Animaniacs' Revived at Hulu With 2-Season Order.*

The deal involved two new seasons, Hulu, Warner Bros. Animation, and Amblin Television—a lot of cooks in that kitchen, which may in part explain why it took so long. Probably a lot of dough, too.

Two seasons of *Animaniacs* were going straight to Hulu, which also got the library rights to *Animaniacs* and *Pinky and the Brain,* another spin-off we did called *Pinky, Elmyra and the Brain,* and the entire *Tiny Toon Adventures* collection.

It seemed like half my life was going to stream on Hulu, a channel that didn't exist, on a platform nobody could have imagined, when we first recorded the show back in 1993. This also meant that the old episodes would be streaming alongside the new version; the first time fans could watch—and, gulp, compare—the two versions.

From the announcement, it was clear Hulu was going to be making a huge investment in the show, which it billed as its "first original series made specifically for families." Craig Erwich, senior VP of content at Hulu, was quoted as calling *Animaniacs* "one of the most beloved, inventive and funny animated franchises in history," and said its "cast of witty characters can live on."

And by cast, he meant the characters, not the voice actors—us, in other words—whose names appeared nowhere in the announcement in the *Hollywood Reporter* or *Variety* or any of the Hollywood trades. Believe me, I checked.

In the end, my fear we'd be replaced with the season nine cast of *The Bachelor* proved ridiculously wrong. The announcement that *Animaniacs* was coming back on Hulu in 2020 was made before we made our deals as voice actors, and so that put a whole different spin on things. Once the show was announced, our agents and lawyers got to work. It was contracts back and forth, redlining, red-penciling, and then we finally got the deal done in about April.

There were only two agents involved. Jess and Maurice are represented by one agency and Tress and I are represented by Sutton, Barth & Vennari. In April 2018, a year after the La Mirada show and almost exactly two years after I started undergoing cancer treatment, the deal for the actors was signed, sealed, and delivered.

I'm not one who usually says things happen for a reason. So much random craziness has accompanied my career that I'm a little more cynical about that. But I submit that this time, at least, fate played a role.

For two years I had gone so nuts over whether the shows were coming back and whether I'd be coming back with them that I lost sight of the fact that, had it happened any sooner, I probably couldn't have done it.

I don't think I really was ready until the middle of 2018. Emotionally I was still getting better. I still had little things that I had used and developed in characters for years that I couldn't do physically as a result of the treatment.

One of the things I couldn't do was this one single silly sound, but one I had come to use frequently. It's a kind of lascivious gurgle, like Roy Orbison makes in "Pretty Woman." You'd be surprised how handy that sound could be.

When I first started going back to work after my treatment, one of the shows on which I had a semiregular spot for a few years was *Curious George* for PBS. In the show there were these critters. I'm not a particularly good animal impressionist, à la Michael Winslow or Frank Welker, but they called upon me to be the voice of a pigeon who's a friend of George's. His name is Compass the Pigeon.

I got the gig because our director, Kris Zimmerman, had heard me—don't ask me where—make that gurgling sound. She thought it sounded like a pigeon cooing.

The first time I did Compass after my treatment, I couldn't get the sound out. Try as I might, I couldn't do that crazy coo. The radiation had physically changed the shape of my throat, and my salivary glands had gone dry. Bottled water didn't help.

So I fudged it. I made the sound in the front part of my mouth instead of way back in my throat as I usually did. The first thing Kris said was, "That doesn't sound the same, Robbie. Are you okay?"

"Oh, I'm good," I said, but I wasn't. She knew what I'd been through, but that wasn't even probably what occurred to her—it was just like, "It doesn't quite sound the same." It needed to sound the same. They had established that sound in earlier episodes. Kids really pay attention to that stuff.

Kris said, "Isn't it maybe a little deeper?"

We worked around it. But the problem weighed on me. I had survived cancer, but I was still less than whole. That little growl was a tool I'd had in my tackle box of audio fly-fishing for years.

It was more than a year later, in March of 2018, when I was messing around the house, and, for whatever reason, out came the sound. It sounds so silly, but being able to do that coo sound the way I had done it before my treatment was a huge deal for me. It was another acknowledgment that I was one more step back to normal.

Anyway, had *Animaniacs* been picked up in January of 2017, when I was still coo-less, I couldn't have done what I do now. I have more sounds at my disposal. I have more notes at the top of my range. I was a different person, then. Emotionally I was different. Now, in every sense of my personal and professional life, I am ready to go.

With this deal in 2018, I was closing a door and opening another one, literally, with a big fat WB logo on it.

Warner Bros. decided to celebrate the relaunch by treating Tress, Jess, Maurice, and me to dinner, serendipitously enough, nostalgically enough, at Morton's. Sam was supposed to be there, but he couldn't make it at the last minute. But the studio was to be represented by executive producer and showrunner Wellesley Wild, producer Gabe Swarr, and Warner Bros. animation executive Audrey Diehl.

I distinctly remember driving to the restaurant, and as I walked in, I took a moment to absorb it all. It was May 2018. We were literally eight feet from where I'd sat at a different table with Randy and Jess and Tress and Sam in 2016. I was thirty-five pounds lighter, and I still couldn't taste the steak I was about to eat. I'd have to down an entire glass of water to swallow one bite of hot sourdough bread.

But what would make the evening taste so incredibly sweet was that it was all behind me. The only thing in front of us was the excitement of working on this show that had brought so much joy to millions of people. And due to the miracles of modern medicine, I was going to be able to enjoy it.

Over the next few weeks, after we signed our deals, the producers gave the voice actors an overview of the show, some general outlines of what we'd be doing. But we didn't get any scripts until July of 2018, a week or so before we started recording.

Reading my lines for Yakko and Pinky, the first ones written in twenty years, was weird in the most wonderful way. The world had changed so much. Everything about the way people consume entertainment has changed. The show is headed for a new platform, new technology, a new generation of fans. People are going to be able to watch the old original *Animaniacs* and brand-new *Animaniacs* side by side in real time.

But it was the same characters and the same core cast and that same winning creative formula. Everybody's healthy. Everybody's alive. Everybody's still doing their gig. It was an incredible experience to see Yakko, Wakko, and Dot, and Pinky and The Brain, in print again, with new scripts with my name on them.

We found out there was going to be a lot of music with a big orchestra again, and we hit it off with the new showrunner, Wellesley Wild. Sam Register had been in our corner from the beginning, and everything he said—*everything* he said—about using us came to fruition.

When Mr. Spielberg and Warner Bros. were pitching the show to networks, each of us got a call from Warner Bros. through our agents asking for high-resolution head shots. We found out later that during the meetings Mr. Spielberg displayed big blowups of Maurice, Tress, Jess, and me to underscore that the original cast would return.

This may not have happened if *Animaniacs* and *Pinky and the Brain* had been rebooted ten years earlier or even five years later. In the last twenty years, we'd done countless conventions and public appearances. The fans came to know the voices behind the characters, and that mattered to them. We were no longer anonymous parts that could be replaced with a celebrity du jour. Fans would see it as the stunt that it was.

When I was done with my treatments in May 2016, the doctors said I would probably want to give myself two years to become myself again. And I'll be damned, I signed on the dotted line for *Animaniacs* in May of 2018. Everything was conspiring to make this happen.

Recording began in the summer. Pulling into the parking lot, here was the Warner Bros. water tower, our fictional home. I saw Maurice and Jess coming from their cars. They were walking together, and it was just this incredibly wonderful, perfect feeling.

God almighty, here we were, two-plus years and thirty-five radiation treatments and eight chemotherapy treatments later, and it was happening. We went to the studio for the first time in two decades, all of us in one place. There was Tress, Jess, Maurice. It was like everybody coming home to Thanksgiving, but it was twenty Thanksgivings before we got together.

I saw new faces, the production made up of young folks who were just kids the first time we did the show back in 1993. Everybody was all shiny and new except for Tress, Jess, Maurice, and me. One young woman started to cry as she told us how she grew up on *Animaniacs*. They were all so excited, relishing the challenge and the pressure of what they were doing. They were, I think, also a bit frightened, or nervous, maybe.

One young man said to me, "Mr. Paulsen, I grew up listening to you."

I did an old-man voice and said, "What? 'Threw up listening to me'? That's no way to talk to your elders."

While I honor and understand that the original staff made Pinky what he is today, I now have this opportunity to work with all these new people, who are coming at it from a completely different headspace. I am so thrilled to be able to have walked both sides of the track. I got to be there at the beginning, and I'm getting to be there again with a new generation of creative minds.

I savor the responsibility of being an example to them. Maybe some of them went against their family's advice in order to pursue show business. I hope that they could call their parents and tell them, "I worked with Rob Paulsen today, and he was the nicest guy," just as I used to tell my parents, "I worked with Dick Van Dyke, and he was the nicest guy," or "I just had lunch with Steven Spielberg, and he was the nicest guy."

When Tress, Jess, Moe, and I finally got in the studio, we were all like little kids. We held hands, our characters would start to speak, and I'd look over at Tress. She had this big, wide smile that said, *Can you believe this?* To be able to share it again with those people—it was just kind of a miracle.

There was also a melancholy. We looked through the glass and didn't see those familiar faces. We didn't have our beautiful leader, Andrea Romano, who has retired. We didn't have those cartoon geniuses Tom Ruegger and Peter Hastings, who have moved on to other projects. We didn't have our recording engineer, a lovely man named Harry Andronis, who has passed away. Our friend Rich Stone, who was the multiple-Emmy-winning lead composer on *Animaniacs*, was gone. He also had died, as had two other directors, Rusty Mills and Liz Holzman.

So it was the four of us.

And man, we fell right into it. It was like somebody had made a Yakko suit for me to walk around in. I slipped into Yakko like it was nothing.

Listening to Tress do Dot and Maurice do The Brain and Jess do Wakko, I closed my eyes and just sat back. I kept shaking my head. I don't know how many times we all said to each other, "I love you so much, I can't believe we're here, we finally made it, we did it. Thank you, Sam, thank you, Steven."

What's that great song, "The Second Time Around"? Love is lovelier the second time around?

Never in a million years had I thought that we would be here, and I was very cognizant of soaking that whole thing up. I learned so much from the cancer experience about focusing your attention, focusing your love and your energy, and taking an extra moment to meet someone's eye when you're talking to them. Don't miss that opportunity to look over to your buddy and pat him on the back and say, *man, you know, I really am so glad to be here with you.* All of that just hit me square in the face as I sat in that recording studio.

Before cancer, I never took my good fortune, my friendships, my family for granted. But I think I took *time* for granted, and time is such an incredible gift.

Through the original *Animaniacs* run, Tress would always sit to my left in the studio. As we returned to the studio to do it again, she found her usual chair as if not a day had passed.

I looked at her and said, "You're probably not going to remember this," and I recounted a recording session exactly like this one, some twenty-five years earlier. We had just started *Animaniacs*. We had a room full of wonderful talent—Billy West, Jim Cummings, Laraine Newman. The script was cracking. The voices flew out of us. I had looked at Tress to my left and said, "It just does not get any better than this."

I was wrong. It can get better than that. This is better.

AFTERWORD
A Session with Dr. Otto Scratchansniff

"My session today is with Rob Paulsen, about whom a book is being written by himself. The book is essentially a memoir, ja?"

"You can say that, though I don't really know that the world needs another celebrity autobiography."

"Let's just hold the phone right there. You use the term celebrity *with respect to yourself?"*

"Well, it's a generic term."

"No, no, no, clearly you chose that word. What makes you think you are a celebrity? I'm just curious, because, you know, that is a very strong word in your context."

"I mean, some people do consider me a celebrity."

"I don't. What have you done that would call you a celebrity? You're an actor?"

"I'm an actor, yes."

"I don't recognize you."

"I provide the voices for animated cartoon characters."

"For whom do you supply the voice, if I could be so bold to be asking you?"

"How about Raphael from the Ninja Turtles?"

"Not familiar."

"Carl Wheezer from Jimmy Neutron: Boy Genius*?"*

"Not familiar."

"You're not gonna believe this, man, but one of the characters for whom I provided the voice a number of times was you."

"What do you mean, me?"

"Well, you. Dr. Otto Scratchansniff. I created your voice."

"Okay. All right. I think we're gonna need a bigger couch, as they say. I have had this voice since I was first on the Animaniacs *in 1993."*

"You want to hear me do it?"

"I'm right here. I'm probably the smartest person with respect to how I sound."

"Okay, check this out: 'Hello, my name is Dr. Otto von Scratchansniff and I...'"

"Wait a minute, wait a minute, that sounds a lot like me."

"Told you."

"No, no, no, no, no, no, don't make me nuts with you. Now I'm starting to get all anxious. I'm wanting to have the little nervous breakdown. Could you move over? I'm gonna lie down on the couch."

———

Dr. Scratchansniff is my animation shrink. Any time I'm considering making a big career decision, I book a session. It usually ends up like this.

I decided to spare him any personal details. The reality is, I'm still far from 100 percent. I can sing again at a professional level, but my voice is stronger in the afternoon and evening. I used to have my agent book me at 9:00 a.m. I'd do some scales to warm up. Now, that's not really the case. I prefer that they book me after two o'clock in the afternoon.

My throat still hurts. In the morning, I have jaw pain. It's not impossible, but it's there, and I have to stretch my jaw out every morning because the treatments compromised the range of motion of my mouth.

I'm still dry as a bone, the salivary glands the biggest casualty of the treatments. There are different medications to enhance saliva production. They haven't seemed to work for me. I heard that there are several clinical studies and trials that I could be involved in. I may try acupuncture.

I'm 142 pounds. That means I've gained only four pounds from my lowest weight. The doctors want me somewhere between 155 and 165 pounds.

I'm trying. I still can't taste a lot of foods. I used to love pizza. Now it does nothing for me. The first bite I get a mouthful of cheesy goodness, then after three or four bites I can't taste it anymore. The nuance of food is also lost. If I have a piece of red meat in my mouth, I can't tell if it's pork, or lamb, or steak. I could maybe detect duck, because it's greasier. But I couldn't tell you the difference between turkey and chicken.

And there is a difference between turkey and chicken. And I like that difference.

A feast now means cottage cheese and mild salsa. I can eat a whole quart of cottage cheese. If only it had more calories.

Because of the scar tissue, my esophagus is narrower. I find myself taking smaller bites and using water all the time. If it becomes really impossible to eat again, I'll do the procedure that stretches my esophagus. Otherwise, I just don't want anybody or anything invading my throat again.

But you know what: if this is as good as it gets, I'm okay with that. I wrote an email to a friend the other day. I said, "You know what? I'm different. I'm changed."

It's not just a taste for some foods that I've lost. I've gotten to a point where I don't suffer fools like I used to. I remember my dad used to always say, "Lead, follow, or get out of the way." Just like Lee Iacocca in those old commercials for Chrysler.

I'm getting close to that—professionally, anyway. My credits suggest a certain willingness to do damn near anything my agents find. Now, that job slump doesn't scare me anymore. I'm not interested in auditioning for every little thing that comes down the pike. It's a little bit frightening, because I'm so used to saying yes to every project that comes my way. I'm not used to saying, "Gosh, I really don't think I'm interested. I don't wanna hurt your feelings. Thank you, but no, thank you."

Now, it's all about the fans. It's all about the laughter. It's all about the characters.

On a Thursday in November 2018, I booked an *Animaniacs Live!* show at the fifteen-hundred-seat Miller Outdoor Theatre in Houston. Along with Randy and me, Tress and Maurice signed on.

I jumped on the plane at LAX. My wife was out of town visiting relatives in North Carolina. Our longtime friend Sandra was staying at our house with our Yorkie, Tala. Tala needed some tender loving care, since we had to put down her sister just a few weeks earlier.

As the plane taxied down the runway, my wife sent me a text message: Had I heard about the brushfire in Chatsworth in the western San Fernando Valley? Our house is located in the hills to the west, about twenty miles away. I looked out the airplane window and didn't see even a wisp of smoke in the distance.

By the time I landed in Houston, my wife had texted to say that a second brush fire had broken out in Newbury Park, about ten miles to the west of our home. My wife's doctor lives with her daughters and a potbellied pig in Newbury Park and faced evacuation. We arranged for all of them to stay out of our house, which seemed far and safe from both fires.

Our home was now occupied by four people, a dog, and a pig. Through Thursday evening I monitored the news online. One of the fires was getting closer to my house. I called the fire station, which is located about a quarter mile from my home, and they said no evacuations had been ordered.

Then at about midnight, I got the call. First responders were cruising through our neighborhood on a bullhorn. Everybody had to get out. Now.

My wife's doctor heard the announcement and woke up Sandra. They all split—the doctor, her daughters, and the pig to other friends, Sandra and our dog to Sandra's house in Hollywood.

I kept calling the fire station. First things looked good. Then early Friday morning they told me the fire had leaped across the 101 freeway and was barreling toward our house.

I decided I was going home. I took an Uber to the airport at 3:00 a.m. for a 6:00 a.m. flight to Los Angeles. Back and forth I went on my phone, texting with my wife, with the fire department, with anybody I could think of who would know what was going on.

Nobody did. I didn't know if my house had survived the fire. The reports were grim. The fire had torn through my area, taking out Malibu Creek State Park and the famous Paramount Ranch movie location, where *Westworld* and countless other shows were filmed.

Finally, the fire department told me that they weren't letting anybody into the neighborhood. Even if I flew back to LA, I couldn't get to within miles of my home, or whatever was left of it. I felt incredibly helpless. I called my wife.

She told me that if there was ever a time for me to follow the old axiom that the show must go on, this was it. At the very least, I could make some money and bring some joy to the audience, and to myself. I rescheduled my flight and headed back to the hotel.

That night, Friday, I performed songs from *Animaniacs*. I had done them before under adverse circumstances—depressed about my career, ravaged by cancer treatments. But none were as surreal as this. Randy, Tress, Moe, and I went through the show as if nothing was happening. I didn't say a word about the fire.

And it was a balm. Audiences do immeasurable things for a performer. You may never fully know what laughter and applause does to the soul if you haven't experienced it yourself. Every time my mind drifted to my house, the audience brought me back. The only way I could pay them back was to do my job and put on a show worthy of the money these folks spent, give them a memorable evening.

The next day, Saturday, I flew home. I spoke to Sandra, who had worked miracles. My wife is a photographer, really world-class, and Sandra had scooped up her work and some of our son's baby stuff and such. That put my wife's mind to rest. Sandra also got other personal effects.

Including my Emmy. She sent me a text with a photo of it.

My neighborhood still remained under an evacuation order. Tress, Jess, Maurice, Randy—everybody offered places for me to stay the night. Instead, I went to my son and daughter-in-law's place in LA, where I spent the night with my dog. (Proud dad aside: My son is a big deal in the gaming world at the YouTube channel GameXplain; fans at Comic-Con now ask me if I'm Ash Paulsen's dad!). Sunday morning I got a room at the Burbank Holiday Inn, since I had to work Monday morning directing *Rise of the Teenage Mutant Ninja Turtles*.

The news reports said the fire had gone through our neighborhood, but I couldn't get a clear answer as to whether my house was spared. When I was in the car, I got a call from my wife from North Carolina. She told me to pull over and look at a video she'd sent me. My brother-in-law, who works for the phone company, managed to get to my street to take a cell-phone video.

The hillside was black. The palm trees were toast. But our house survived. It was the first time I could breathe easy in days.

I drove up the freeway, and when I got to my turnoff, police stopped me and asked for my identification. They told me I could go to my house, but I could only spend ten minutes there. The concern now was looters, and the cops were trying to keep the number of people in the burn area to a minimum.

I was able to get to my house. It stood there, unscathed. But when I opened the front door, it reeked. Before the fire we had refinished the floors. The house smelled like a combination of floor-refinishing compound and smoke. Amazingly, the electricity worked. I turned on fans and aired it out.

My fire insurance covered a hotel, but most of the places nearby were booked for days with other evacuees. It just so happened, however, there were vacancies in the local luxury hotel, the Four Seasons. And they took dogs. So Tala and I would tough it out in a well-appointed room with high-thread-count sheets and a minibar.

Fire does not discriminate. The hills and canyons where I live do have their share of celebrity homes that you saw in the news. But they're also filled with longtime residents who bought when it was cheap decades ago. The Four Seasons parking lot reflected this, with Rolls-Royces parked next to clunkers.

Like everybody else in the lobby of the hotel, I was wearing a particle mask. (Which I happened to have in the car with my earthquake kit. Life in LA.) The acrid smoke still hung heavy in the air, and my radiated throat was vulnerable. As I checked in, I yanked off my mask and made the standard joke: if this is struggling during a disaster, I'll take it.

The young folks behind the counter asked me if my home was okay. I said it was. They asked me if I had just come from work, and I said, yes, and they asked where I worked, and one thing led to another, and pretty soon I was talking like Carl Wheezer. Like I've said before, it happens.

That's when I noticed the family behind me, a woman with her two young boys. The mom looked absolutely exhausted and disheveled. Clearly she'd been crying.

"Sorry, I don't mean to intrude," she told me. "We couldn't help but overhear you, and I have to say, this is the first time my children and I have laughed in the last three days."

It was the most incredible compliment I'd ever received. I knew it was not me that made them smile. It was the characters. It reminded me of how powerful these little creations are. Moments like this have happened so many times—and have only increased since Randy and I hit the road with our show and after the announcement of the return of *Animaniacs*.

I posed for selfies and did some more voices—the boys were big *Turtles* fans—and watched them get on the elevator, one of the boys on his phone, clearly googling me, for he told his brother, "He's *that* guy."

But after everything that had happened over the last two years, the feelings seemed magnified. It was a slap in the face, a reminder of how much could have gone wrong and didn't. I have learned more about being a human being in the last two years than in the previous sixty.

I'm a better person. I'm a better father, a better husband, a better friend. And I'd argue I might be a better actor, because I can access parts of myself that I'm only now willing to share with people. Who would have thought that to do a better job at making people laugh, I had to learn to cry?

It reminded me how lucky I was to be in show business, how lucky I was to be there, that day, at that hotel, with those good people. It reminded me how lucky I was to be alive.

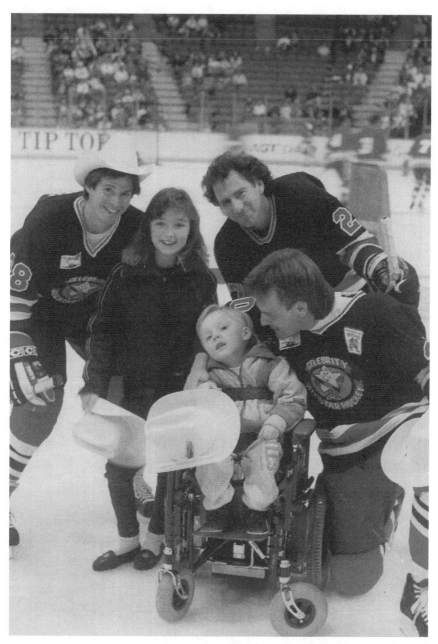

My brave little Turtle buddy, Chad Gozzola, surrounded by love. L-R: Ken Olandt, Jen Gozzola, his sister, Jerry Houser, and yours truly, moments before I quietly broke down as I started to grasp what "Turtle Power" was all about. Little did I know how much Chad and his family would inspire me to be courageous in my own fight for life 26 years later. Thank you, Gozzolas, for letting me into your hearts. An impossibly perfect gift. Calgary Saddledome. February, 1990.

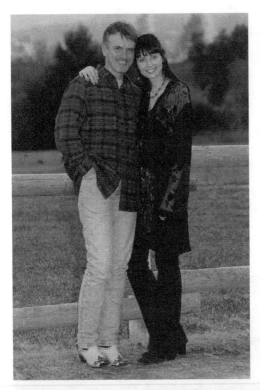

Parrish Todd. My wife. A gifted photographer, world class Mom, and a daily reminder that strength, class, kindness, and beauty, inside and out, are not mutually exclusive. EVERY base was covered during my tap dance with cancer. With Ash and me, she's had to put up with boy germs for a LOOONG time.

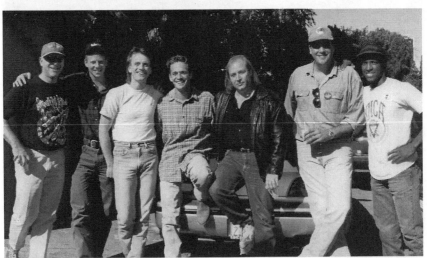

The *Biker Mice From Mars* creators and a few cast members. L-R: Rick Ungar, Ian "Vinnie" Ziering, "Throttle", Luke Perry, Tom Tataranowicz, Brad "Greasepit" Garrett, Dorian "Modo" Harewood. SO much fun and frankly, I've got my mousey little fingers crossed for a reboot. I seem to play a lotta mice. ROCK 'N RIDE, CITIZENS!!! Studio City, California. 1995.

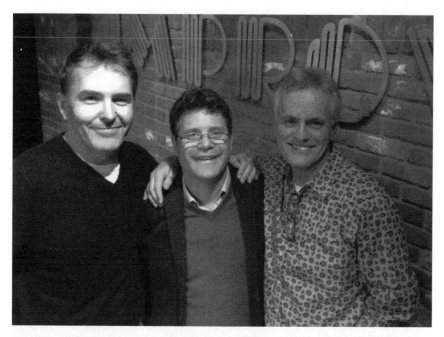

3 Raphaels at The Improv for a "Talkin' Toons Live" show. L-R: Nolan North, Sean Astin, and the OLD-(est) Raphael. Photo courtesy of James Cluster. Hollywood. 2015.

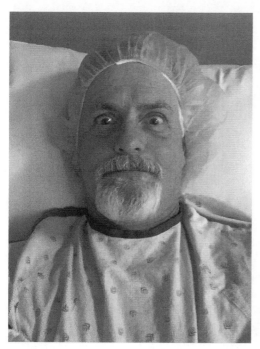

Does this hospital bonnet make me look freaked out? First biopsy after my diagnosis. I was joking with the nurses before I went under. When I awoke, the first face I saw was my boy's. I was really hurting, but Ash's strength and love were exactly what I needed. Los Angeles. February, 2016.

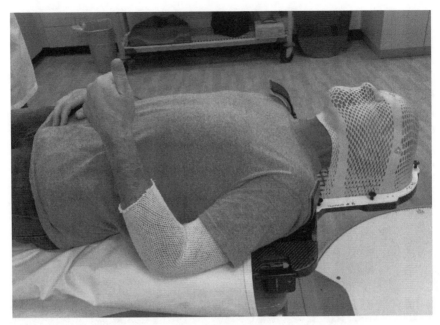

Locked and loaded. Let's light this candle! West Hills, California. March 21st, 2016.

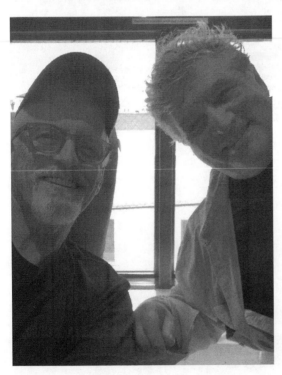

Pinky and The Brain at one of Pinky's chemo treatments. Maurice LaMarche is a truly gifted actor, sure. So are a lotta folks in Hollywood. Far more important are Moe's humility, empathy, and kindness. Not sure whether he'll ever take over the world, but his friendship's taken over my heart, and I'm a better man as a result of his example. Selfie, Beverly Hills. April, 2016.

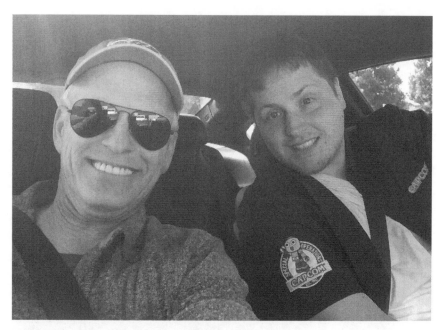

My boy driving the old man to my final radiation treatment! May 5th, 2016.

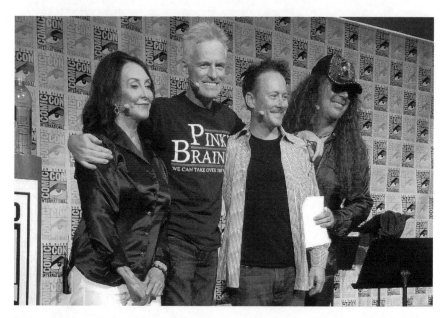

Back at my happy place: onstage with my *Animaniacs* brothers and sister. L–R: Tress "Dot" Mac-Neille, me, Randy Rogel, and Jess "Wakko" Harnell. Probably too soon for me, and yet not soon enough. Forty-plus pounds lighter and just starting to get used to "Rob 2.0." Still am, as of this writing. Photo courtesy of my Turtle brother, Townsend Coleman. San Diego Comic Con. July, 2016.

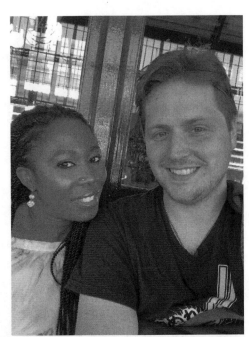

The pride and joys of my life: my daughter-in-law, Abisola, and my son, Ash. Kind, beautiful, smart, talented...my son is too.

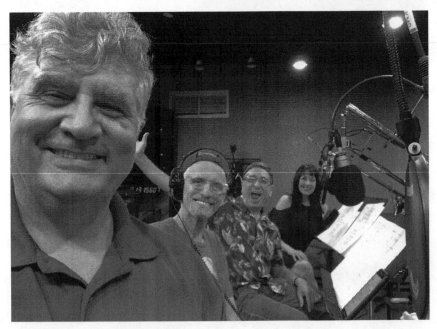

Maurice, me, Corey Burton, and Grey DeLisle at a "Pinky and The Brain" recording session for the new Hulu version. I've had the pleasure of Corey and Grey's friendship for 40 years and 25 years respectively. Jackpot. Warner Brothers Animation. Selfie, early 2019.